ACKNOWLEDGEMENTS

To my father, and farmer, Ned Harle, thank you for everything you've done for me. Your quiet confidence and hard-working nature never went unnoticed. Much of this book is a result of your tutelage. I would be remiss if I didn't also thank my mother, the woman beside the farmer, Sherri Harle. I love you both.

A special thanks goes out to my incredible wife, researcher and editor, Denise Harle; without her, this book would not have been thought of. Also, to my father-in-law, Robert Mayo, and cousin, Jamie Horowitz, thank you for your sharp eyes and helpful minds; your editing was greatly appreciated.

TABLE OF CONTENTS

INTRODUCTION

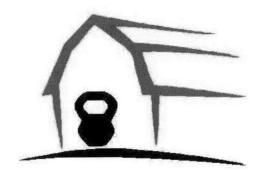

"I BELIEVE HARD WORK AND HONEST SWEAT ARE THE BUILDING BLOCKS OF A PERSON'S CHARACTER..."

- A FARMER'S CREED

INTRODUCTION

WHY DID WE CREATE FARMER GYM'S ALMANAC?

Born and raised a farmer's son, I began to understand the value of hard work and the importance of a strong, healthy body at a very young age – a farmer's livelihood depends on these principles. It was there, on the farm, where I learned that nothing is given; it's earned. A person's fitness mirrors the philosophy of a farmer's labor; just as farmers build, grow, and shape the land through abundant effort, people build, grow, and shape their bodies through dedicated discipline. Farmer Gym itself, and Farmer Gym's Almanac, were created to share the principles of hard work applied to total-body fitness, and to empower people to use any environment as a gym.

The workouts you'll find in this Almanac are based on a variety of isometric, isotonic, and higher-intensity approaches that employ your body as the machine. The result is a combination of elevated heart rate and strengthened muscles – and well-rounded fitness from head to toe. Unlike other almanacs, Farmer Gym's Almanac will never be outdated, because the information within is rooted in sound physiological maxims. Our hope is that you will use the Almanac year after year.

WHO IS THIS BOOK FOR?

Plainly put, this book is for *anyone* and *everyone* who desires to advance their health and wellness through exercise. More specifically, this book is for YOU if you meet any of the following criteria:

- You can't seem to find time to get to a gym

INTRODUCTION

- You are bored with your exercise regimen and are looking for a change in your workouts
- You can't afford a gym membership or home gym equipment
- You are new to working out but want to develop a doable workout regimen
- You just don't like the "feel" of a gym
- You prefer to exercise outdoors
- You desire privacy when you're exercising
- You are constantly on the go (or on the road) and need a flexible workout program
- You want the benefits of a personal trainer – specific instructions and a variety of workouts – without the expense
- You stay at home with your children and need workouts that can be done in your house
- You can't stand doing traditional cardio
- You desire total-body fitness with workouts that can be done in less than 30 minutes

HOW DO YOU USE THE ALMANAC?

In the spirit of the Farmer's Almanac, we have included 365 days of workouts. And, as with any reference book, Farmer Gym's Almanac is meant to be consulted as a resource as appropriate and not necessarily read and implemented from cover to cover. Just as you wouldn't pick up a dictionary and read it front to back, you aren't to perform Farmer Gym's Almanac workouts 365 days in a row each year. Instead, use Farmer Gym's Almanac like this: *Make it your own.* Indeed, the very fact that the Almanac is a reference book is exactly why it is for everyone.

INTRODUCTION

Make the Almanac your own, to create a workout plan that suits your needs, likes, abilities, and schedule. There are a few ways to do this:

Skip Around. The workouts in the Almanac are listed in no particular order. Feel free to skip around, selecting workouts that interest you or that challenge you in particular ways. The Index is searchable by the name of each exercise and by the body parts worked by each exercise, allowing you to easily tailor your exercise program to fit your goals and preferences.

Scale. Built into each workout are mechanisms for making the workout more or less challenging. You can increase or decrease the number of repetitions you perform. You can increase or decrease the number of rounds you perform. You can increase or decrease the amount of rest between rounds or sets. You can also modify certain exercises to increase or decrease the difficulty (e.g., perform Incline Push-ups on your knees to make the strain on your chest muscles less intense). Don't be afraid to kick up the intensity if you find that you aren't breathing heavily or feeling any exhaustion during the workouts.

Rest. Everyone using this book should take rest days. Beyond that, you can utilize the number of rest days to advance your particular fitness goals. Those interested in significant weight loss or muscle growth may choose to perform these workouts 5 or 6 days a week, while those simply desiring more basic exercise for mental health or fitness maintenance may perform workouts only 3 days a week.

In addition to complete rest days, you should rest particular muscle groups, so that you are not overtraining them. Muscles need time to recover in order to grow and develop in a healthy way. When you are exercising on consecutive days, select your workouts so that you are working different muscle groups. If your chest muscles are sore from yesterday's Staggered Push-ups, then choose a workout that doesn't tax the chest today. Again, the Index will be helpful for you here, as it lists which body parts are challenged by each exercise and workout.

Rest within workouts is instrumental, too. Take as many seconds of rest as you need during these workouts in order to safely perform the remainder of a set, round, or the next round. Never push yourself without resting, at the expense of good form or breathing. It's always better to take a break and recover than to burn out and quit, or to lose your form and injure yourself.

Track Your Progress. Each workout in the Almanac includes its own Notes section, where you can take notes about your performance and measure your progress over time. This will serve to help you not only learn about your body, but also be encouraged as you see your performance improve on the various exercises. If competition motivates you, then make it a competition against yourself, and keep score.

Work. Our final and perhaps most important tip is this: Work. Don't shortchange yourself when everything you need for improving your fitness is literally at your fingertips (assuming you are holding this with your hands as you read). You'll get out of this book what you put in. So, work – and then reap what you sow.

INTRODUCTION

REALLY? NO EXERCISE EQUIPMENT?

Farmer Gym's Almanac is a body-weight workout book. For the many people who are accustomed to traditional gym workouts, the absence of exercise equipment may not only be foreign but also even dubious. Well, don't take our word for it; try it yourself and see. You *will* strengthen and tone your muscles if you challenge yourself with the Almanac's workouts.

The one type of body-weight exercise Farmer Gym employs that does require a simple piece of equipment is the Pull-up/Chin-up. For the Pull-up/Chin-up, you will need a basic high bar or rod. More than likely, you live near a park or schoolyard with a suitable bar. If not, or if you'd prefer to perform the Pull-up/Chin-up workouts at home, you can purchase a portable bar for as little as $25.

And if you just can't stand the thought of letting your dumbbells and ankle weights collect dust – or if you work your way up to a point where you could benefit from an extra challenge in these Almanac workouts – you may incorporate light hand weights and ankle weights as you wish.

WHAT'S WITH THE KETTLEBELL WORKOUTS?

As you may have already noticed, there are 50 Kettlebell workouts in the final section of the book – and, no, these are *not* entirely body-weight workouts. For those who already like working out with Kettlebells, the Kettlebell Section is simply a bonus offering in the Almanac. But the primary reason Farmer Gym has included this selection is to introduce people to the benefits of Kettlebell workouts. Farmer Gym is hoping to acquaint

INTRODUCTION

you with Kettlebell workouts and perhaps expand your exercise horizons and help you change up your workouts even more. Here's why:

The Kettlebell is great for building strength, power, stability, and cardiovascular endurance. Due to its weight and changing center of gravity during use, the Kettlebell requires the body to exert force and maintain balance in a number of positions. Compared to large, fancy machines, the Kettlebell is very inexpensive – plus, it can be stored out of the way and takes up very little space. The best part about the Kettlebell? It can go anywhere.

How to choose the correct weight: Always err on the side of caution, and don't attempt to increase the Kettlebell weight too quickly. Start with a lower weight and gradually increase the size of the Kettlebell you are using. It's important to perform each exercise correctly before moving up in weight. Many professionals recommend that females start with a weight between 15 and 25 pounds, gradually increasing to 35, 45 pounds, and so on. It's recommended that males start with a weight between 25 and 35 pounds, gradually increasing to 45, 55 pounds, and so on.

CAN YOU REALLY GET FIT WITH 20-MINUTE WORKOUTS?

The workouts in the Almanac are all in the 20-minute range – some a little less, some slightly more. This might surprise you, or even make you skeptical. But research has shown that vigorous exercise sessions lasting just 20 minutes are very effective in achieving fitness results. This kind of high-intensity workout has been found to improve cardiovascular health, increase fat burning, and boost energy levels. And, because Farmer Gym's Almanac workouts are designed to use a high number of repetitions to take the muscles to fatigue, these workouts tear down the muscle fibers, which leads to muscle toning, strengthening, and hardening. Trust us, and see for yourself. Twenty is plenty.

If you find that the 20-minute workouts become easy, go ahead and incorporate an extra round or add a repetition or two, to stretch it out a few more minutes. Conversely, if you find that the 20-minute workouts feel too difficult, exclude a round or take away a repetition or two, to subtract a few minutes; then work your way up.

A WORD ON NUTRITION

A substantial part of health and wellness lies in proper nutrition. When an exercise regimen is adopted in conjunction with a healthful diet, the results are synergistic. Although nutrition is beyond the scope of this book, Farmer Gym emphatically encourages healthy eating, and we work with our clients to provide them with counseling on the kind of nutrition that can help them more effectively achieve their fitness goals. If you are seeking science-based nutritional guidance to maximize your results from using Farmer Gym's Almanac, find out more at http://farmergym.com/coaching/online-training-option-1

THE FINE PRINT

Farmer Gym's Almanac does not contain medical advice. As with any exercise program, you should consult your physician before using Farmer Gym's Almanac if you face any of the following risk stratifications: have any pre-existing situations that include but are not limited to a heart condition, pain in your chest from physical activity, dizziness or loss of consciousness when working out, known bone or joint problems, or are taking prescription drugs. In addition, see your physician if you are female over age 55, a male over age 45, have a family history of heart disorder, have been a cigarette smoker in the past half-year, have led a sedentary life, are considered obese, are hypertensive, have high levels of lipids in your blood, or have a form of diabetes or other metabolic disorder. Likewise, when you are performing the Almanac workouts, if you experience unusual pain, or if something doesn't feel right to you...STOP. Getting fit does not require injuries!

Although Farmer Gym has structured the workouts in the Almanac to avoid unhealthy muscle strain through overtraining, there remains an extremely unlikely chance of muscle damage from overuse. If you begin feeling pain in your joints or experience unusual soreness or health issues, temporarily discontinue your exercise regimen and see a medical expert.

Results are not guaranteed. How much progress you see toward your fitness goals will depend on how often you exercise, how hard you push yourself while exercising, what your diet consists of, your genetic composition, how active you are apart from working out, and other factors. Working out with the Almanac is an excellent start but is not the only determinant of your health and fitness outcome.

INTRODUCTION

Be smart. Stay hydrated by drinking water before, during, and after your workouts. Work out in a place that is a safe temperature. And if you begin feeling dizzy or light-headed, stop.

One more thing. It's important to conduct your workouts in places that allow for stable footing. Make sure your exercise location accommodates safety, by choosing a flat, even surface that is not slippery or rocky.

You must be 18 years of age to use Farmer Gym's Almanac, and Farmer Gym is not liable for any injuries resulting from use or misuse of the Almanac.

Enough with the disclaimers. Let's start growing hard bodies!

THE EXERCISES

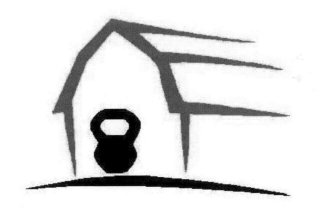

"TAKE CARE OF YOUR BODY. IT'S THE ONLY PLACE YOU HAVE TO LIVE."

— JIM ROHN

THE EXERCISES

This section of the Almanac contains detailed descriptions of how to perform each exercise included in the Almanac's workouts, accompanied by photographs for illustration. If you find that you need additional illustration, you can view video demonstrations of each exercise in Farmer Gym's online Video Library at http://farmergym.com/library/. The Farmer Gym Video Library is accessible for free and is compiled from YouTube clips that provide accurate examples of proper form.

In most of the exercise descriptions below, you will see instructions to keep your spine straight and your core tight while performing the exercise. Your "core" consists of your abdominal muscles in your mid- to lower torso, which you should tighten by engaging the muscles. Similarly, keeping your spine straight requires awareness of aligning your vertebrae (or back bones) from your neck all the way down to your tailbone, without rounding your back or arching it. We may also refer to this as a "neutral" spine. Keeping your spine straight and core tight is very important for protecting against injury, so we flag it upfront here and repeat it throughout the exercise descriptions.

Warm-up and Cool-down. Before beginning each workout, spend up to 5 minutes getting your heart rate up and your blood flowing through your muscles. You can do this by jogging or marching in place, walking briskly for a short distance, or doing some Jumping Jacks.

When you complete each workout, spend a few minutes slowing your heart rate gradually by marching in place again or walking around the block, and then stretching.

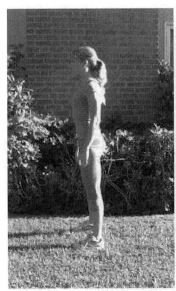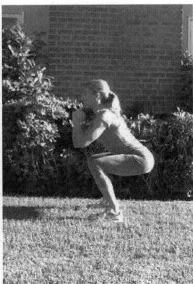

AIR SQUAT

* Stand with your feet at shoulder width and toes pointed slightly outward
* Keep your chest up, back straight, and core tight
* Descend by pushing your hips and gluteus back and down
* Keep your weight on your heels
* Stop once your thighs are parallel to the ground
* Ascend by pushing through your heels
* Finish the squat in the starting position, standing up straight
* Your knees should not travel forward past your toes, nor should they turn inward
(Scaled: Perform while supporting yourself with a wall or fixed structure)

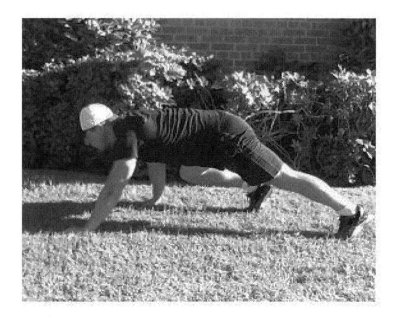

BEAR CRAWL

* Place both feet and hands on the ground while facing the ground
* Place your hands under your shoulders
* Keep your hips low, and maintain a tight core
* To travel, bring one hand and its opposite foot forward
* Continue this alternating process, by moving one hand and its opposite foot forward

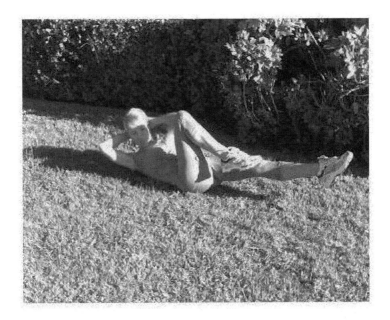

BICYCLE

* Lie on your back with your knees up and at approximately a 90-degree angle and feet off the ground
* Place your fingertips behind your head and keep your shoulders off the ground
* Twisting your torso while maintaining a tight core, bring one elbow toward its opposite knee, and draw the knee in until they meet
* Meanwhile, fully extend the other leg so that it is straight and a few inches off the ground
* The elbow not brought in should point away from your body
* Continue this process by alternating your elbow to meet its opposite knee

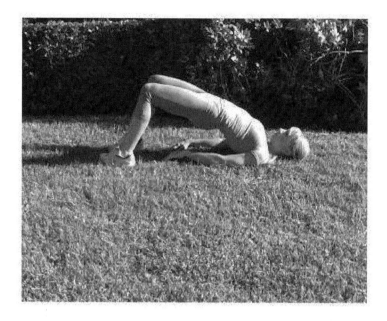

BRIDGE

* Lie on your back with your feet on the ground at hip width and knees at a 45-degree angle
* Place your arms along your side, engage your core, and squeeze your shoulder blades together
* Pushing through your heels, lift your hips off the ground, toward the sky, and squeeze your gluteus
* Lower your body in a controlled manner to the starting position

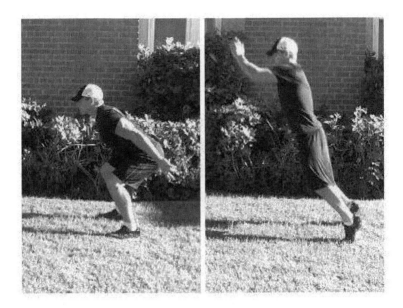

BROAD JUMP

* Stand with your feet at hip width and toes pointed forward
* Keep your chest up and core tight
* Reach your arms back behind your body as you descended to approximately the half-squat position
* Explode forward by jumping from the balls of your feet
* Land with your weight somewhat forward

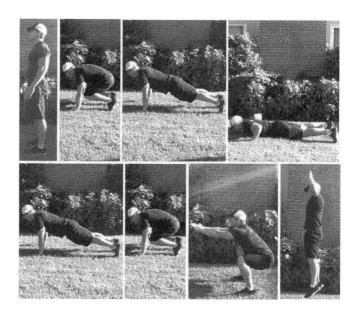

BURPEE

* Stand with your feet slightly wider than shoulder width
* Keep your chest up and core tight
* With the weight on your heels, squat down and place your hands on the ground
* With the weight on your hands and shoulders, jump and extend your body until you are in a Plank-like position
* Descend until your chest touches the ground
* Ascend to the Plank-like position by straightening your arms, and jump your knees forward to your chest
* Squat up, jump up into the air, and land in the starting position
(Scaled: Perform the Push-up portion from your knees)

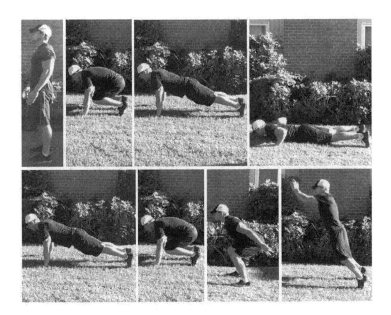

BURPEE BROAD JUMP

*After performing the Burpee (described above),
immediately perform the Broad Jump (described above)
(Scaled: Perform the Push-up portion from your knees)

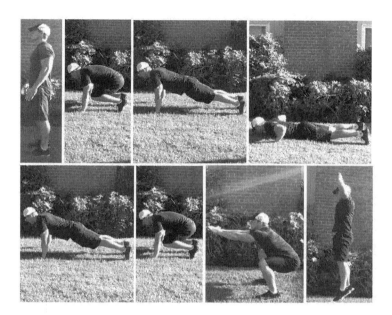

BURPEE PUSH-UP

* While performing the Burpee (described above), perform the Push-up (described below)
* Instead of descending your chest to the ground once, as in the basic Burpee, descend your chest twice, to include the extra Push-up
(Scaled: Perform the Push-up portion from your knees)

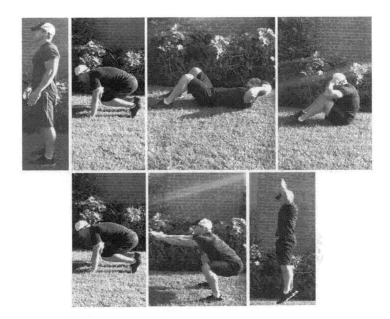

BURPEE SIT-UP

* Begin performing the Burpee (described above)
* From the bottom of the squat, instead of jumping back into the Plank-like position, quickly sit down, lie on your back with your knees bent and feet on the ground, and perform the Sit-up (described below)
* From the top of the Sit-up, jump up into the air, and land in the starting position

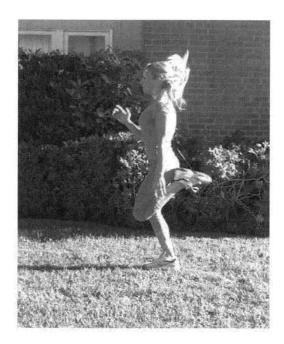

BUTT KICK

* Stand with your feet underneath your hips
* Keep your chest up and core tight
* Bring your heel straight back and bend your knee, bringing your heel toward your gluteus
* As your heel contacts your gluteus, your opposite arm should move forward in a running-like motion
* Lower your heel to standing, and alternate legs with this heel-to-gluteus motion

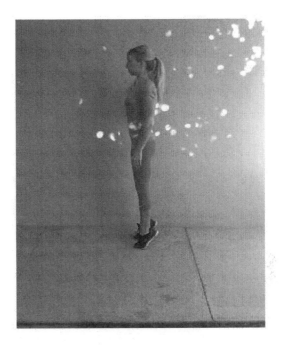

CALF RAISE

* Stand with your feet underneath your hips
* Keep your chest up and core tight
* Push through the balls of your feet until you are on your toes
* Lower your heels to return to the starting position

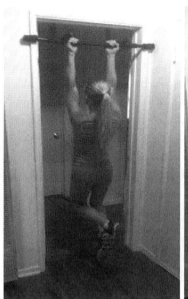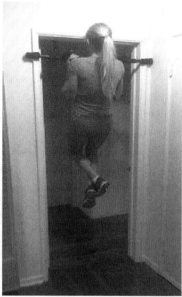

CHIN-UP

* Hold the bar at approximately shoulder width with your palms facing towards you
* Keep your core tight, spine straight, and shoulder muscles contracted
* Your head should be in line with your spine
* With both arms extended above you, pull your body up in a controlled manner until your head is near bar level
* Upon reaching the top, slowly lower your body to the starting position, with arms again extended
(Scaled: Perform by hanging from the bar in the start position for time, engaging your shoulder and upper back muscles; or, perform a flexed-arm hang, or partial chin-up, and slowly lower your body to the start position)

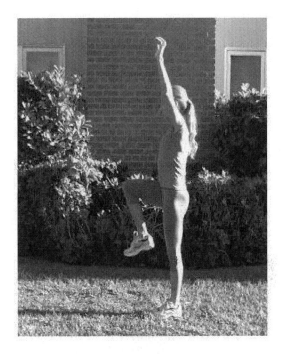

CLIMBER

* Stand with your feet underneath your hips
* Keep your core tight and spine straight
* Raise one knee to approximately 90 degrees and your opposite arm toward the sky
* Repeat this pattern, with alternating leg and opposite arm reaches

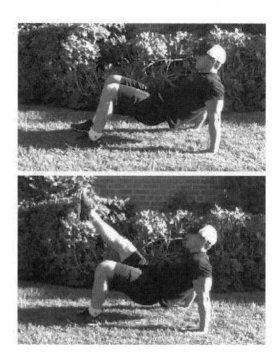

CRAB KICK

* Place both feet and hands on the ground while facing the sky, and lift your core
* Your feet should be approximately hip-width apart, pointing forward, with knees slightly bent
* Your hands should be slightly wider than and behind your shoulders, pointing away from your body, with your elbows slightly bent
* With your hips off the ground, kick one leg into the air while both arms are holding your body stationary
* Repeat this pattern, with alternating leg kicks

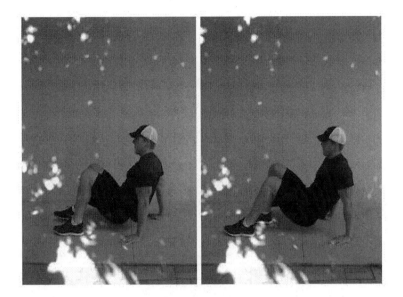

CRAB WALK

* Place your body in the same position as the Crab Kick (described above)
* Instead of kicking your legs, walk your feet and arms backwards by alternating each leg and its opposite arm

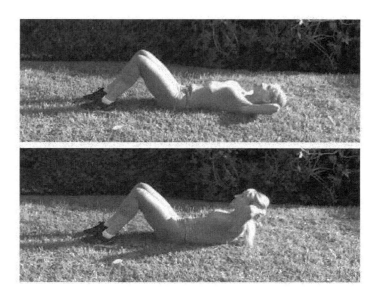

CRUNCH

* Lie on your back with your feet on the ground at hip width and your knees at a 45-degree angle
* With your elbows out and wide, place your fingertips behind your head and pull your shoulder blades together
* While tightening your abdomen, raise your torso off the ground
* Once you have reached eye level to your knees, lower back down in a controlled manner until your shoulders touch the ground
* Avoid bringing your chin to your collarbone, rounding your back, or arching your back

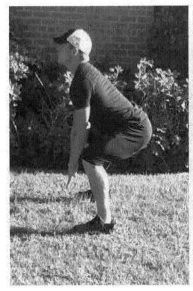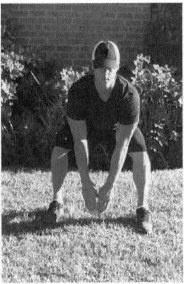

DEADLIFT

* Stand with your feet at approximately shoulder width and toes pointed slightly outward
* Keep your chest and chin up, and keep your head aligned with a straight spine throughout the exercise
* Bend your hips and knees at the same time
* In a controlled manner, continue to bend your knees and shift your hips back and down
* Your shoulders should remain upright and straight as you lower toward the ground, and will be over your knees at the bottom position
* Your knees should not travel forward past your toes, nor should they turn inward
* Once you reach the bottom position – with your fingertips 6" from the ground or less – stop
* While maintaining a tight core, push your body up through your heels
* Ascend to the starting position by simultaneously straightening your knees and hips

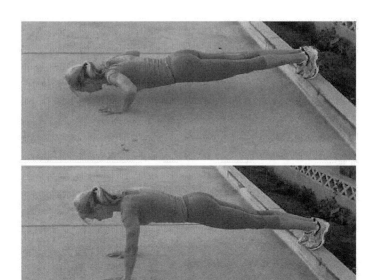

DECLINE PUSH-UP

* Begin in a Plank-like position, with your feet at about hip width and mounted on a stable elevated surface, such as a staircase
* Place your hands wide enough on the ground to form a 90-degree angle with your elbows
* While maintaining a tight core and straight spine, lower yourself to the ground, or within 6" from the ground, and then raise yourself to the starting position

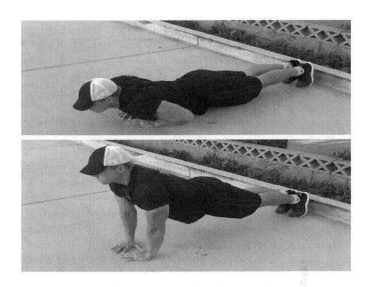

DIAMOND PUSH-UP

* Begin in a Plank-like position described below), with your feet slightly closer together than hip width
* Place your hands close together, forming a diamond shape between your thumbs and forefingers
* While maintaining a tight core and neutral spine, lower yourself to the ground, or within 6" from the ground
* As you descend, keep your elbows in close to your torso and bring the center of your chest toward your hands
 * Upon reaching the bottom, press up to the starting position
(Scaled: Perform from your knees)

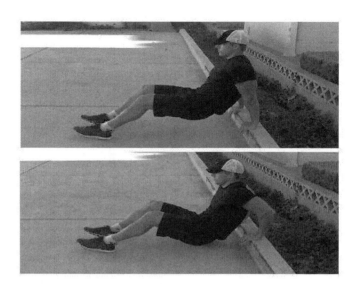

DIP

* Place your heels on the ground and your hands on a stable elevated surface (or on the ground), while facing upward
* Your feet should be just inside hip width, with your knees slightly bent
* Point your hands forward while placing them behind your gluteus and slightly wider than your hips
* While maintaining a tight core, press through your hands and heels, pushing your hips and gluteus off the ground, by bending and extending your elbows
* Continue this up and down motion

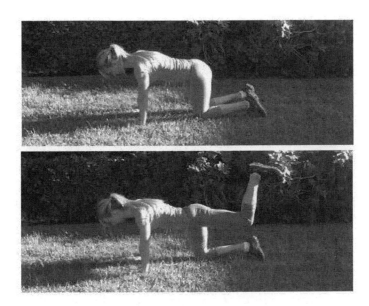

DONKEY KICK

* On all fours, place your hands under your shoulders and knees under your hips
* Maintain a flat back and tight core
* Bring one leg in toward your torso then extend it backwards and upwards toward the sky
* Raise your leg until the knee is bent at a 90-degree angle, with your foot parallel to the ground
* Repeat this process by alternating legs

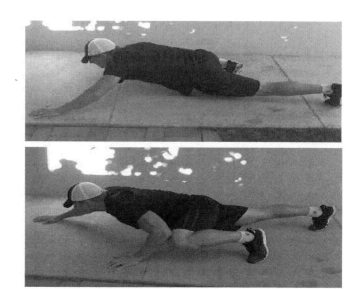

DRAGON WALK

* While on all fours, knees and elbows bent, and body kept low to the ground, place your weight on your hands and toes
* While tightening your core, pull one knee forward and the same side's elbow backward until both touch
* The opposite side's hand should be extended, with your foot trailing behind your body
* Continue moving forward by repeating this alternating process

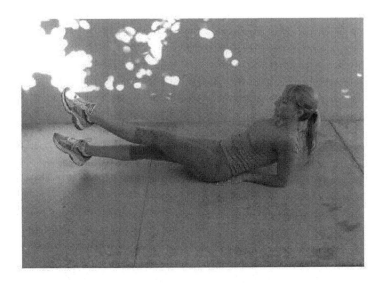

FLUTTER KICK

* Lie on your back with your hands placed under your gluteus, with your palms down
* Tighten your core and extend your legs, holding them a few inches off the ground
* Lift one leg to approximately a 45-degree hip angle while holding the other stationary, keeping both legs straight
* Lower the elevated leg to the starting position, while lifting the other leg to a 45-degree hip angle, and continue alternating legs in this manner

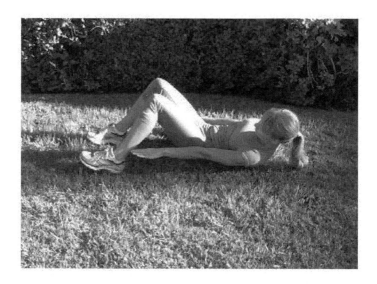

FOOT-TO-FOOT CRUNCH

* Lie down on your back with your hands at your sides, knees bent, and feet on the ground at hip width or slightly narrower
* Slightly raise your shoulders and head off the ground so that your core is tightened
* With your stomach muscles engaged, lean your torso to one side and touch your heel with the fingertips of your hand on the same side as the heel
* Return to the starting position, keeping your shoulders and head elevated, and complete the same movement on the opposite side.
* Avoid bringing your chin to your collarbone or rounding your back

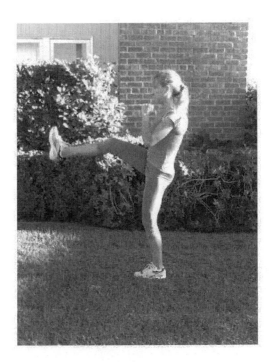

FRONT KICK

* Stand upright with your arms bent and held out in front of your body, and your elbows close to your rib cage
* Clench your hands in a fisted, defensive position
* While maintaining a tight core and upright spine, lift one leg, knee first, and extend it to just above waist level
* Return the leg to the ground and repeat the process with the other leg

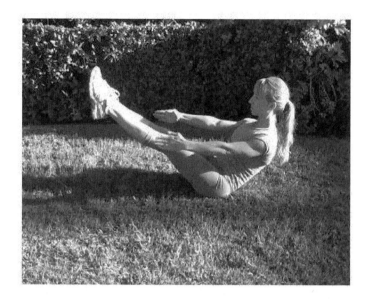

FROZEN V SIT

* Begin in a seated position, with your torso and feet both extended in the air to form a V shape with your body
* Although they won't touch your feet, reach your arms toward your feet
* Maintain a tight core and straight spine
* Hold this position for the allotted time

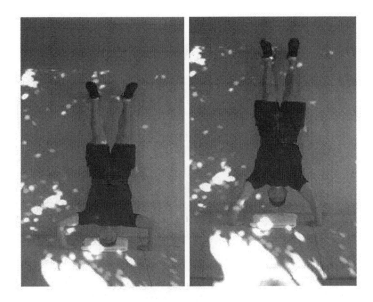

HANDSTAND PUSH-UP

* Before attempting to perform this, be certain you are confident and strong with Pike Push-ups
* Against a wall, push or kick your body upside down into a handstand position, with your heels against and your face away from the wall
* With your hands shoulder-width apart, bend your elbows and slowly lower the top of your head, with your chin slightly tucked, down to the ground (onto a towel or small pillow)
* Once you reach the bottom position, push yourself up until your body is fully extended in a handstand
* Keep your core tight and body close to the wall throughout the exercise
(Scaled: Perform the Pike Push-up; or, perform the Walk Walk)

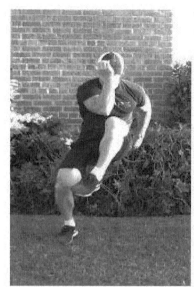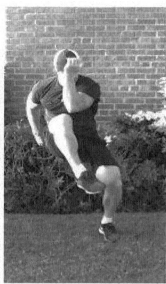

HEISMAN

* Stand with a slight knee bend and arms at your sides
* Start by bringing one knee up toward your chest and your opposite elbow toward your knee
* With the leg that is on the ground, push off, hopping laterally toward the side with the lifted knee
* Gently land approximately 12" – 18" wider than where you started
* The leg that pushed off the ground should now be up, with the opposite elbow reaching for the raised knee
* Maintain a tight core throughout the workout

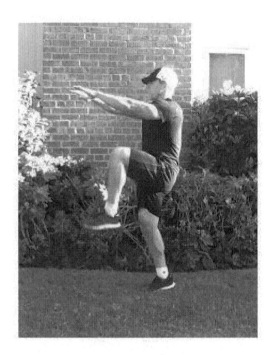

HIGH KNEE

* Stand with your feet hip-width apart
* While on the balls of your feet, start by bringing one knee up toward your chest while raising your arms straight out in front of you (or, raise only your opposite arm, with a bent elbow, in a running-like motion)
* Your knee should reach at least hip level
* Bring your leg back to the ground and repeat this process on the other side, keeping your arms straight out in front of your chest

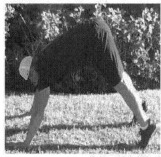 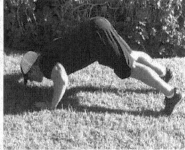

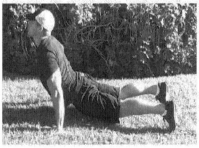

HINDU PUSH-UP

* Begin in a Plank-like position, placing your weight on your hands (which should be at approximately shoulder width) and toes
* Move your gluteus toward the sky to a point where your body is an inverted V – your arms and back are aligned, legs are in a straight line, and your eyes are looking backwards at your feet
* While bending your elbows, bring your hips down and torso forward
* Before your head reaches the ground, start arching your back (with your core tightened) so that your face is looking towards the sky
* Straighten your arms, and return to the starting Plank-like position

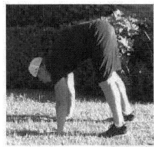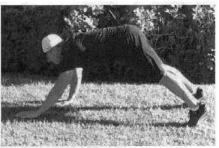

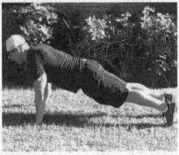

INCHWORM

* Stand with your feet pointed forward, hips bent, torso toward the ground, and hands in contact with the ground
* Walk your hands forward, with your heels eventually rising from the floor
* Continue walking forward until you reach the Push-up/Plank position
* Once you reach the Push-up/Plank position, start walking your feet forward toward your hands, taking short steps without moving your hands

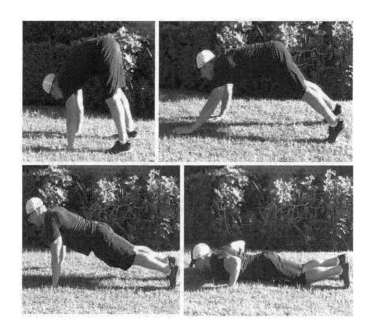

INCHWORM PUSH-UP

* While performing the Inchworm (described above), perform the Push-up (described below)
* Once you reach the Push-up/Plank position, perform a Push-up, then continue to finish the Inchworm
(Scaled: Perform the Push-up portion from your knees)

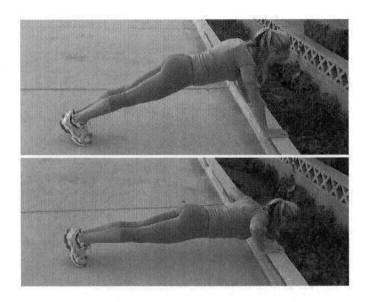

INCLINE PUSH-UP

* Place yourself into an inclined Plank-like position, with your feet on the ground at about hip width and your hands securely gripping a staircase or other elevated stationary surface
* Place your hands wide enough on the elevated surface to form a 90-degree angle with your elbows when at the bottom of the Push-up
* While maintaining a tight core and neutral spine, lower yourself to within 6" of the ground, and then raise yourself to the starting position by straightening your elbows
(Scaled: Perform from your knees)

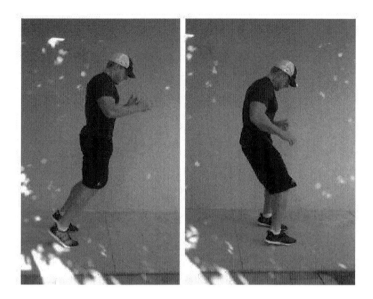

JUMP-OVER

* Stand with your feet hip-width apart, knees slightly bent, and arms at your sides
* While standing behind an obstacle, such as a piece of tape or other jumpable object, bend into a quarter-squat position
* Explode through your hips and calves to jump over the object, landing softly on the balls of your feet
* In the same motion you jumped forward, jump backward over the object to the starting position

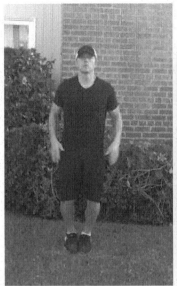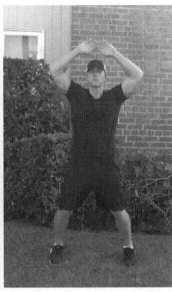

JUMPING JACK

* Stand with your feet together and arms at your side
* With a slight jump, spread your feet apart to shoulder width
* During the jump, stretch your arms out and up in a wave-like manner until your hands touch above your head
* Return to the starting position by simultaneously jumping your feet back together and sweeping your arms out and down to your sides

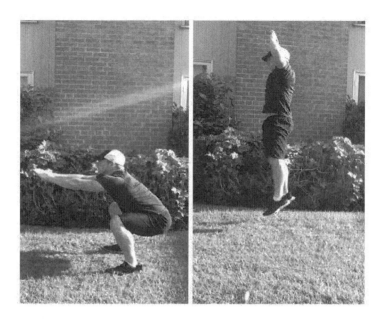

JUMP SQUAT

* Stand with your feet hip- to shoulder-width apart and toes pointed slightly outward
* Keep your chest up, spine straight, and core tight
* Descend by pushing your hips and gluteus back and down
* Keep your weight on your heels
* Briefly stop once your thighs are parallel to the ground
* Explode by pushing through your heels then rolling onto the balls of your feet, and jump into the air
* Softly land on the balls of your feet with your knees bent and feet underneath your hips, and absorbing the force of the landing with your hips

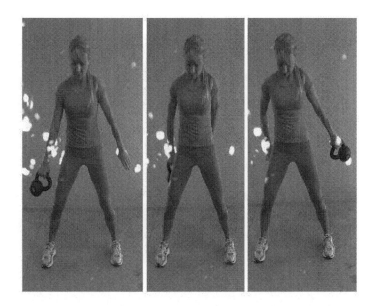

KETTLEBELL AROUND THE WORLD

* With a slight knee bend, stand with your feet at about shoulder width and your arms at your side (while holding the Kettlebell with one hand)
* Start by passing the Kettlebell around your body near waist height
* At approximately the center of the body, both front and back, pass the Kettlebell to the opposite hand
* Although your body will likely sway some, retain a rigid posture and attempt to prevent your body from swaying substantially

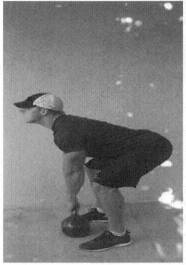
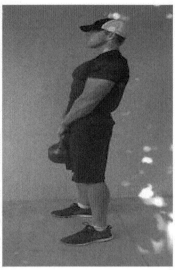

KETTLEBELL DEADLIFT

* Stand with your feet at shoulder width or slightly wider and toes pointed slightly outward
* Place the Kettlebell under your body, in between your legs
* Lift your chest and chin, and keep your chest up and head aligned with a neutral spine
* Bend your hips and knees at the same time
* In a controlled manner, continue to bend your knees and shift your hips back and down
* Your shoulders should remain straight as you lower toward the ground, and will hover over your knees at the bottom position
* Your knees should not travel past your toes or bend inward
* At the bottom, grab the Kettlebell with two hands
* While maintaining a tight core and stable spine, ascend by simultaneously straightening your knees and hips and pushing through your heels until you are standing up straight

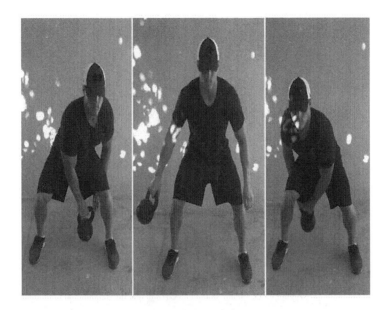

KETTLEBELL FIGURE-8

* Stand with your feet slightly wider than shoulder width and toes pointed slightly outward
* Place the Kettlebell in between your feet and slightly ahead of your body
* Lift your chest and chin, and keep your head aligned with a neutral spine
* Bend your knees slightly while pushing your gluteus back and out as you bend over to grasp the Kettlebell
* While maintaining a tight core and straight spine, hold the Kettlebell in one hand and swing it through your legs, catching it between your legs with your other hand from behind your body
* Go back and forth, around both legs, from front to back, repeating this alternating release-and-catch action

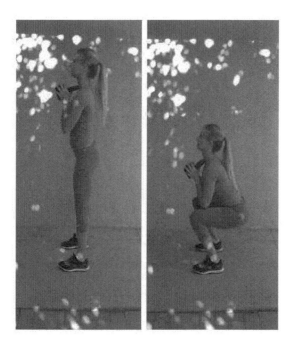

KETTLEBELL FRONT SQUAT

* Stand with your feet at shoulder width and toes pointed slightly outward
* Grab the Kettlebell by the handle, and hold it close to your chest with your elbows in
* Keep your chest and chin up, spine straight, and core tight
* Descend by pushing your hips and gluteus back and down
* Keep your weight on your heels
* Stop once your thighs are parallel to the ground, without letting your knees go past your toes or turn in
* Ascend by pushing through your heels
* Finish the squat in the starting standing position

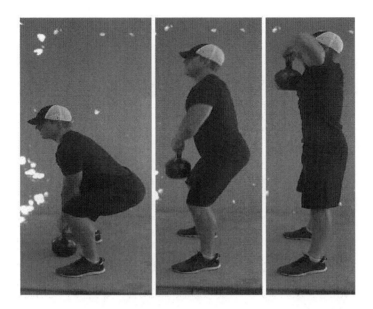

KETTLEBELL HIGH PULL

* Stand with your feet wider than shoulder width and toes pointed slightly outward
* Keep your chest and chin up, spine straight, and core tight
* Descend by pushing your hips and gluteus back and down, without letting your knees go past your toes or turn inward
* Keep your weight on your heels
* Grab the Kettlebell as you push through your heels and ascend to the top; at about midway, pull the Kettlebell up toward your chin
* Keep your elbows held high once the Kettlebell reaches chin level
* Return to the ground by reversing the way in which you ascended

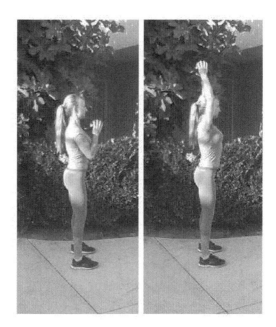

KETTLEBELL MILITARY PRESS

* Stand with your feet hip-width apart
* Grab the Kettlebell by the handle, and hold it close to your chest with your elbows in
* Hold your wrists straight and keep your elbows tight to your body
* With a tight core and straight back, drive the Kettlebell up and over your head, as you straighten your arms
* In a controlled manner, reverse the action, and return the Kettlebell to the starting position

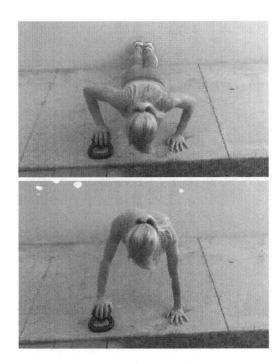

KETTLEBELL PUSH-UP

* Lie face down on the ground with your feet closer than hip width
* Extend your arms in front of you, in line with your shoulders, with one hand on the ground and one hand on the Kettlebell
* With your toes on the ground and your elbows close to your side push through your hands until your arms are extended
* At the top of the push, release your hand from the Kettlebell and walk your opposite hand over to the Kettlebell and assume the up position you were just in
* Return to the ground by slowly by bending your elbows until your chest reaches the ground
(Scaled: Perform from your knees)

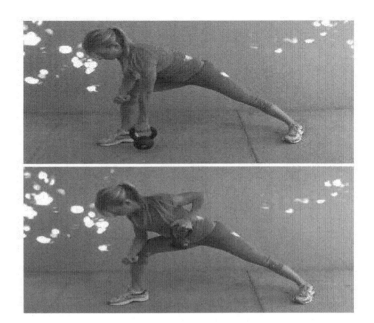

KETTLEBELL ROW

* Stand leaning forward, with one leg in front of the other and feet spread far apart
* Your front leg should be bent, and your front knee should not be past your toes
* Your gluteus should be back, and your rear leg should be slightly bent and facing forward
* The arm not engaged in the lift should rest on the front knee
* With your free arm, grab the Kettlebell and lift your shoulder first, then your elbow, until the Kettlebell has reached your torso
* Gently lower the Kettlebell back to the ground as you picked it up

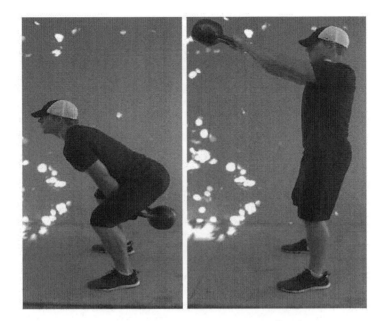

KETTLEBELL SWING

* Stand with your feet approximately shoulder-width apart and toes pointed slightly outward, with the Kettlebell on the ground between your legs
* With your chest up and knees slightly bent, push your hips back, and keep your weight on your heels
* Pull the Kettlebell close to your body and let it travel between the inside of your thighs
* Pop your hips and swing the Kettlebell forward
* Clench your gluteus when your hips are open
* Let the Kettlebell use momentum and reach eye level
* Your arms should stay loose as the Kettlebell travels back to the start position

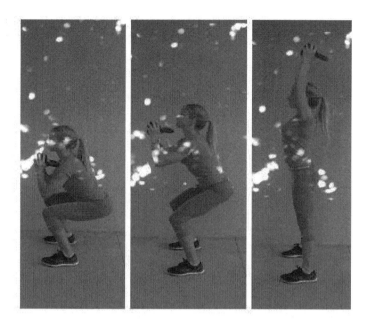

KETTLEBELL SQUAT PRESS

* Stand with your feet at shoulder width and toes pointed slightly outward
* Grab the Kettlebell by the handle, and hold it close to your chest with your elbows in
* Keep your chest and chin up, spine straight, and core tight
* Descend by pushing your hips and gluteus back and down
* Keep your weight on your heels
* Stop once your thighs are parallel to the ground, without letting your knees go past your toes or turn inward
* Ascend by pushing through your heels
* With your momentum, continue to drive the Kettlebell up and over your head, and lock your elbows out
* In a controlled motion, descend to the Kettlebell Front Squat starting position

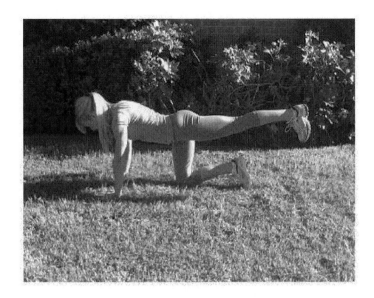

KICKBACK

* Begin in a Plank-like position, with your hands under your shoulders and your knees under your hips
* Maintain a flat back and look forward
* Bring one leg in toward your torso then extend it straight backwards, until it is parallel to the ground
* Bend and lower the straightened leg so that you are back on your hands and knees, and alternate legs

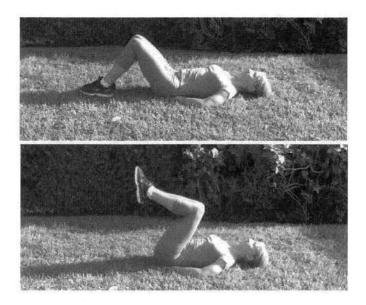

KNEE LIFT

* Lie with your back and feet on the ground, with your knees bent at approximately a 45-degree angle
* Place your hands under your lower back and gluteus
* With your feet together and knees bent, raise both feet off the ground and bring your knees toward your chest
* Continue this movement until your hips are off the ground and knees are over your chest
* Reverse the movement to return to the starting position

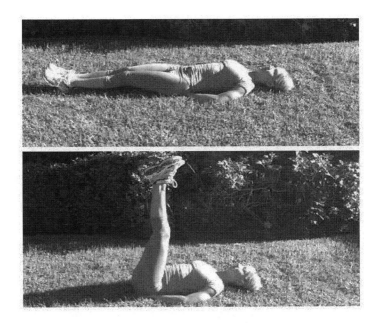

LEG LIFT

* Lay with your back and legs on the ground
* Place your hands under your lower back and gluteus
* With your feet together and legs straight, raise your legs off the ground and bring them up until your toes are above your torso
* Slowly lower your legs until they are approximately an inch from the ground
(Scaled: Perform the Knee Lift)

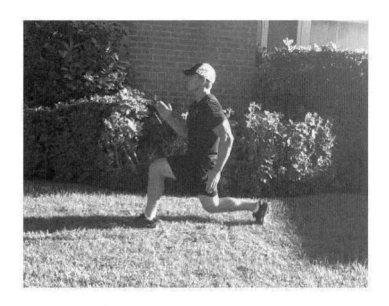

LUNGE

* Stand upright with your feet together
* In a controlled manner, lift one leg off the ground and forward
* Take a step, land with your heel first and foot pointing forward, and slowly shift the weight of your body onto your forward leg
* Maintain an upright torso, tight core, and straight spine
* Continue forward until your thigh is parallel to the ground, without letting your knee go past your toes
* Once in the lunge position, push off the front leg and return to the starting position, and alternate legs
(Scaled: Perform while supporting yourself with a wall or fixed structure)

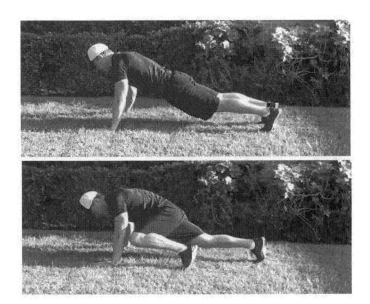

MOUNTAIN CLIMBER

* Begin in a Plank-like position, with your toes and hands on the ground
* Place your hands slightly ahead of your shoulders, with your fingers pointed forward
* Keep your hips low, back straight, and core tight
* Squeeze your shoulder blades together and down your back
* Bring one knee forward and toward your chest, with your foot touching down on the ground underneath your torso, while bracing yourself on the toes of your extended leg
* With your hands on the ground and upper body engaged, jump to switch leg positions

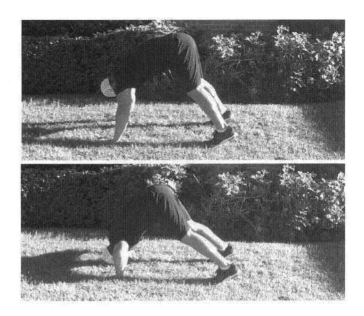

PIKE PUSH-UP

* Stand with your feet wider than shoulder width, hips bent and torso forward, and your hands on the ground underneath your shoulders
* Your legs should be straight, gluteus in the air, and upper body pointed toward the ground
* Your head should be between your arms
* Bend your elbows and slowly bring your head to the ground, where you will end by looking backwards through your legs
* You should be on the balls of your feet when your head is touching the ground
* Once at the bottom position, push yourself away from the ground until your arms are extended and you are back in the starting position
(Scaled: Perform from your knees)

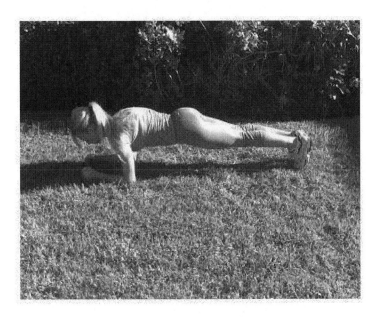

PLANK

* With your body face-down, support your weight on the palms of your hands, or forearms, and your toes
* Your legs should be approximately hip width, and your body should be in a straight line from your head to your feet
* Your shoulders should be aligned over your elbows
* Your head, neck, and spine should be in a straight line
* Keep your core tight
(Scaled: Perform from your knees)

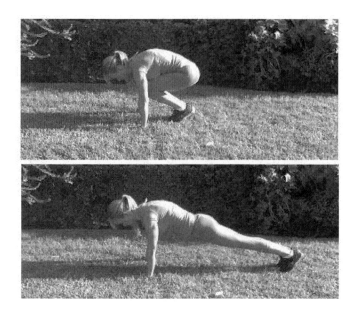

PLANK JUMP

* Begin in a Plank position
* Jump your feet forward as close as possible to your hands, and then jump back to the starting position

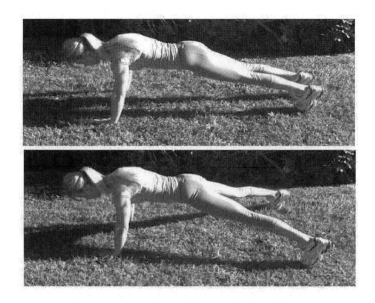

PLANK JUMPING JACK

* Begin in a Plank-like position, with your feet on the ground at about hip width and your arms directly over your hands at approximately shoulder width
* While keeping your upper body stable, begin doing Jumping Jacks with only your legs

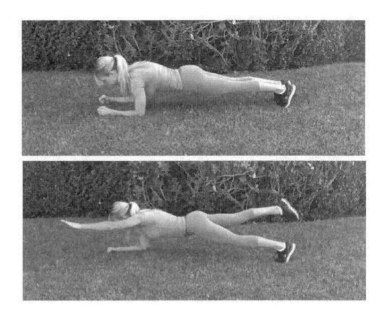

PLANK REACH

* Begin in a Plank-like position
* Lift one arm and its opposite leg off the ground, stretching your hand and foot away from your body
* Maintain a straight line through your lifted arm and leg
* Switch sides and repeat the motion
(Scaled: Perform from your knees)

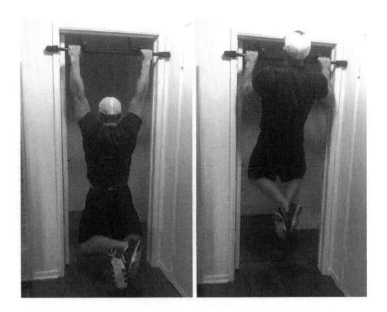

PULL-UP

* Hold the bar with your palms facing away from your body
* Keep your core tight, spine straight, and shoulders engaged
* Your head should be in line with your spine
* With both arms extended above you, pull your body up in a controlled manner until your head is near bar level
* Upon reaching the top, slowly lower your body to the starting position
(Scaled: Perform by hanging from the bar in the start position for time; or, perform a flexed-arm hang, or partial pull-up, and slowly lower your body to the start position)

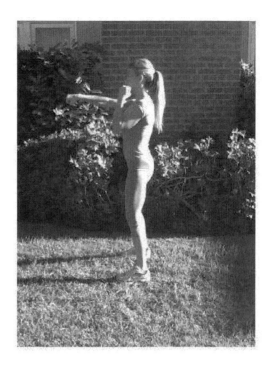

PUNCH

* Stand with your feet hip-width apart
* Clench your fists and keep your elbows bent and by your side
* With a tight core and straight back, drive one arm forward in a punching motion, striking the air at approximately the chest level
* Retract your arm to the starting position and repeat with your other arm

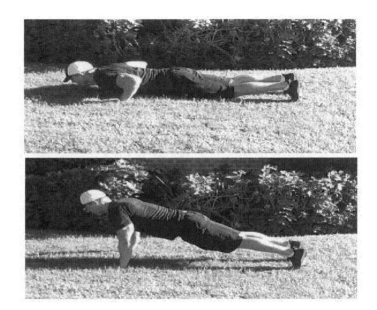

PUSH-UP

* Lie face-down on the ground with your feet at a closer than hip-width distance
* Place the palms of your hands flat on the ground, close to your shoulders
* With your toes on the ground and your elbows close to your side, push through your hands until your arms are extended
* Return to the ground slowly by bending your elbows until your chest reaches the ground
(Scaled: Perform from your knees)

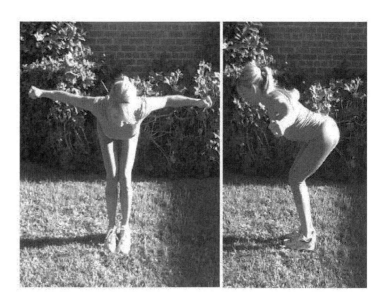

REVERSE FLYE

* Stand with your feet at shoulder width
* With your head up, bend slightly at your knees and move your torso forward toward your upper thighs by bending at your waist and keeping your spine straight
* Your elbows should be slightly bent, with your arms hanging under your chest
* Squeezing your shoulder blades together, raise your arms out to your sides until they are parallel to the ground
* Slowly lower your arms back down by reversing the motion

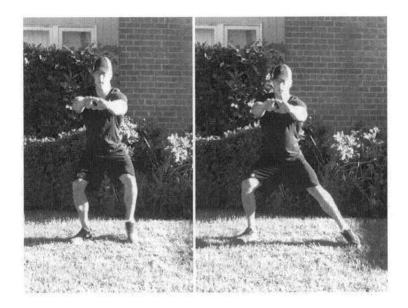

SHUFFLE

* Stand in a quarter-squat position with your feet slightly wider than shoulder width and your chest up
* While on the balls of your feet, move to the side by pushing off one leg and pulling with your other leg
* Your pushing leg should step to where your pulling leg was, as your pulling leg establishes its new position to the side
* Point your toes forward, and don't drag or cross your feet as you move
* Your elbows should be bent and arms held up slightly throughout the exercise

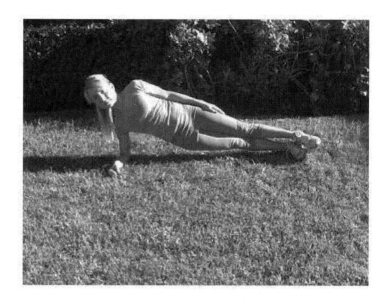

SIDE PLANK

* While on your forearm and outer ankle, lie on your side in a straight line from head to toe
* Your elbow should be directly under your shoulder and your feet stacked on top of each other
* Keep your hips up off the ground, and your head in line with your spine
(Scaled: Perform from your hip)

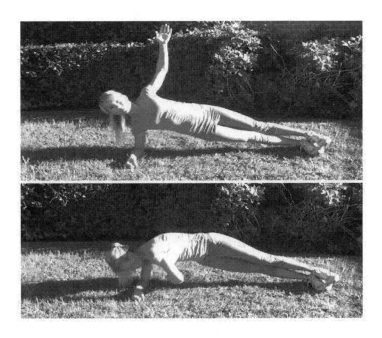

SIDE PLANK TWIST

* While on your forearm and outer ankle, lie on your side in a straight line from head to toe
* Your elbow should be directly under your shoulder and your feet stacked on top of each other
* Keep your hips up off the ground, and your head in line with your spine
* Raise the arm that is not on the floor, and place that hand behind your ear or straight up toward the sky
* Slowly rotate through your torso and touch your upper arm to your lower hand, then return to the starting position
(Scaled: Perform from your hip)

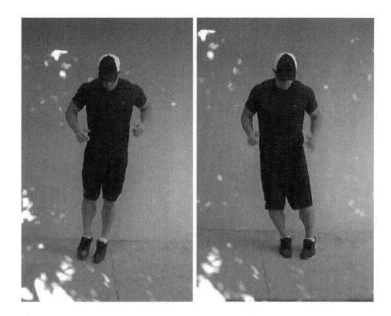

SIDE-TO-SIDE HOP

* Stand with your feet at hip width, your knees slightly bent, and your hands up beside your waist or rib cage
* Select a mark on the ground to jump over
* By pushing through the balls of your feet, hop from side to side over the mark, lifting both feet at the same time and landing on both feet at the same time

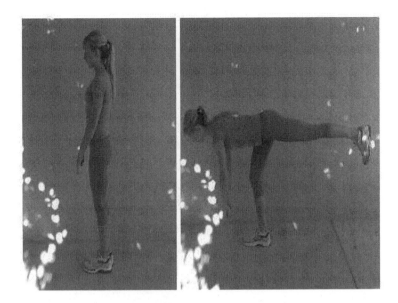

SINGLE-LEG DEADLIFT

* Stand with your legs close to each other
* One foot should be slightly off the ground while the other leg is stationary with a very slight knee bend
* While balancing on one leg, begin to bend forward at your hips
* Maintain a tight core, and keep your back straight and head aligned with your spine
* With the weight on the center of the balancing foot, continue bending forward with your arms hanging toward the ground
* Attempt to straighten your back leg and lift it at the same speed that your torso tips forward, so that it is parallel to the ground
* Return to the starting position by reversing the motion (Scaled: Perform while supporting yourself with a wall or fixed structure)

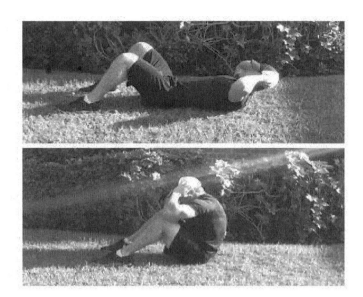

SIT-UP

* Lie down with your knees bent and feet on the ground at hip width or slightly narrower
* With your elbows out and wide, place your fingertips behind your head and squeeze your shoulder blades together
* With your gluteus and feet remaining on the ground, engage your stomach and raise your torso off the ground in a controlled manner until you have reached your thighs with your torso
* Descend by reversing the motion
* Keep your chin up and back straight
(Scaled: Perform the Crunch)

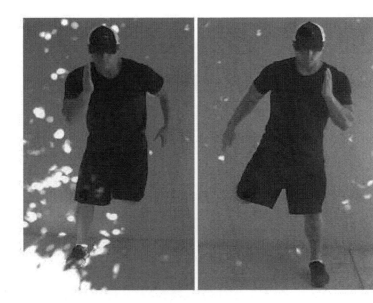

SKATER

* Stand with your feet at shoulder width, bend your knees, and lean over slightly
* Keep your chest and chin up
* From one leg, hop laterally to the other foot, absorbing the force of the hop through your bent hips and knees, and staying on the balls of your feet
* The trailing leg (the one that pushed off) should come close to your landing heel but not touch the ground
* Swing your arms to help maintain your balance
* Continue this process back and forth, alternating legs

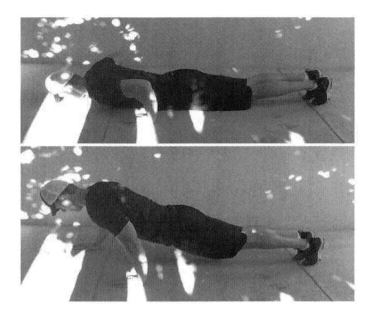

STAGGERED PUSH-UP

* Lie face-down on the ground with your feet closer than hip width
* Stagger your hands, with one forward at approximately shoulder level and the other back at approximately stomach level
* Both hands should point forward
* With your toes on the ground and your elbows close to your side, push through your hands until your arms are extended
* Return to the ground slowly by bending your elbows until your chest reaches the ground
* Alternate hand positions
(Scaled: Perform from your knees)

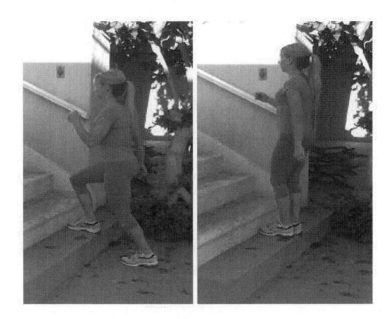

STEP-UP

* You will need a small step, such as a stair on a staircase
* Stand with your feet at hip width
* Keep your chest up
* Push through the ball of one foot, lifting up your opposite knee and placing that foot on the step
* Once your leading foot is securely on the step, bring your other foot to the same step
* If you're performing on multiple steps, such as on a staircase, progress in this manner as you move up the stairs
* Carefully step your trailing leg back to the original position on the ground, followed by the leading leg
* Alternate and repeat process

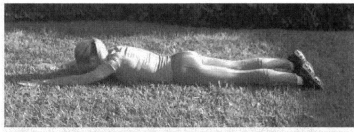
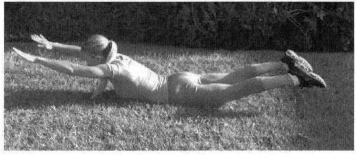

SUPERMAN

* Lie on your stomach with your head straight, arms forward, and feet pointed away from your body
* Raise your arms and legs at the same time by squeezing your upper back and gluteus, careful not to overarch your lower back
* Lower your arms and legs to the ground by reversing the motion
(Scaled: Perform by raising only your upper or lower body)

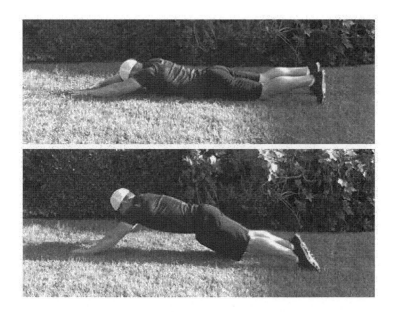

SUPERMAN PUSH-UP

* Lie on your stomach with your head straight, arms forward, and feet pointed away from your body
* Your arms should be at approximately shoulder width and your feet at hip width
* While on your toes, push through your hands, which are extended ahead of you, and raise your body off the ground
* Lower slowly to the starting position by reversing the motion
(Scaled: Perform from your knees)

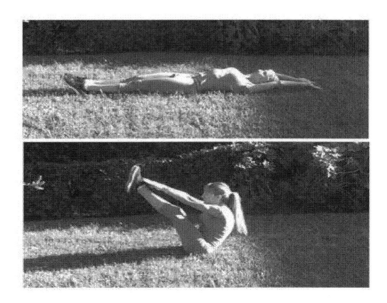

TOE TOUCH

* Begin by lying on your back with your legs and arms extended
* While contracting your abdominals, reach your arms toward your feet
* Maintain a tight core and straight spine
* Once your hands reach, or come close to, your toes, return to the starting position

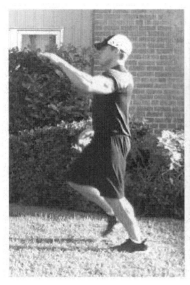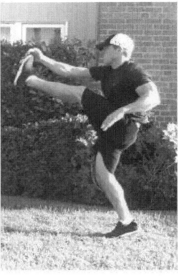

TOY SOLDIER

* Stand with your feet at shoulder width and your arms at your sides
* With controlled movements, kick one leg up in front of you, keeping the other leg on the ground, and reach toward your extended foot with the opposite arm
* Only kick as high as you can – don't strain your leg or knee
* Lower your leg to the ground and then alternate legs and arms

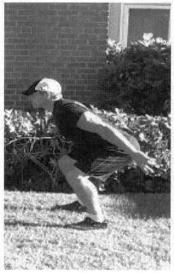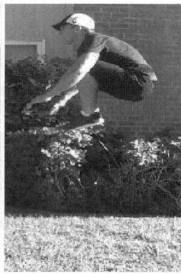

TUCK JUMP

* Stand with your feet at hip width and toes pointed forward
* Keep your chest up and core tight
* Reach your arms down as you bend at your hips
* After you descend to approximately the half-squat position, extend your arms up and jump straight into the air
* While in the air, tuck your knees into your chest
* Land on the balls of your feet, with your knees bent, weight somewhat forward, and chest up
* Immediately spring back into the air and repeat the motion

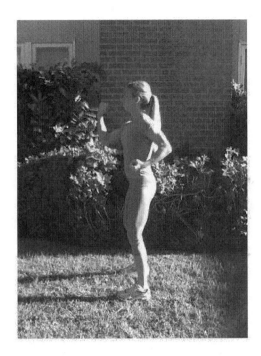

UPPERCUT PUNCH

* Stand with your feet hip- to shoulder-width apart
* Clench your fists and keep your elbows in close to your torso and bent at a 90-degree angle
* With a tight core and straight back, drive one arm up and forward in a punching motion, striking the air at approximately eye level
* Retract your arm to the starting position and repeat with your other arm

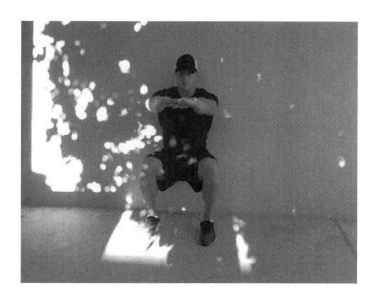

WALL SQUAT

* Stand with your feet at shoulder width and toes pointed slightly outward
* Keep your chest up, spine straight, and core tight
* With your back against a wall, descend by pushing your hips and gluteus back and into the wall
* Keep your weight on your heels
* Stop once your thighs are parallel to the ground, and hold this position
* Once you have reached your allotted time, ascend by reversing the motion
* Your knees should not travel forward past your toes

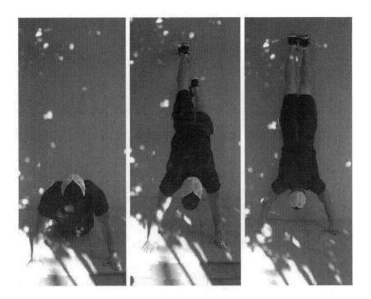

WALL WALK

* Lie face-down on the ground with your feet against a wall
* Push your body off of the ground, and, in a walking motion, move your hands toward the wall and your feet up the wall
* Once you are inverted in a reverse Handstand Push-up position, return to the ground by walking your hands out and feet down the wall, until you are in the starting position
(Scaled: Perform the Pike Push-up)

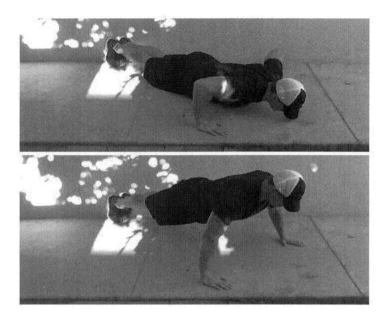

WIDE PUSH-UP

* Lie face-down on the ground with your feet closer than hip width
* Place the palms of your hands flat on the ground, a few inches wider than your shoulders, with your fingers pointing forward
* Bend your elbows to lower your chest to within 6" of the ground
* With your toes on the ground and your elbows at 90-degree angles, ascend by pushing through your hands until your arms are extended
* Return to the ground by slowly bending your elbows until your chest reaches the ground
(Scaled: Perform from your knees)

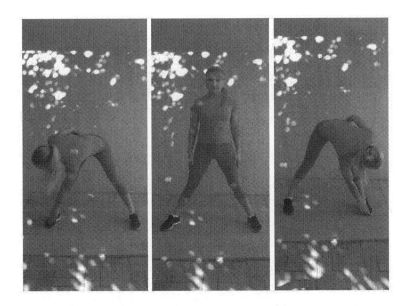

WINDMILL

* Stand with your feet wider than shoulder width, toes pointed slightly outward, and arms at your sides
* Maintain a tight core, keep your shoulders back, and keep your back straight, with your head aligned with your spine
* Slightly push your hips and gluteus out, and carefully bend over to touch one foot with the opposite hand
* The other arm should be by your side or pointing toward the sky with the elbow extended
* Return to the starting position by reversing the motion, and alternate sides

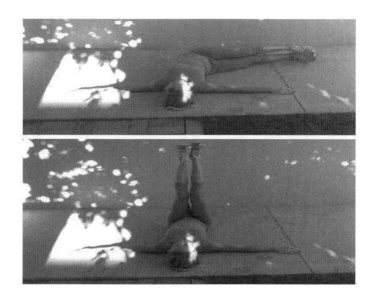

WIPER

* Lie flat with your back on the ground
* Place your arms out to the sides at shoulder level
* With your feet together and legs straight, raise your legs until they are perpendicular to the ground
* From this point, keeping your legs straight, rotate your hips from side to side, lowering your feet close to, but not touching, the ground

365 Days Of
Body-Weight Workouts

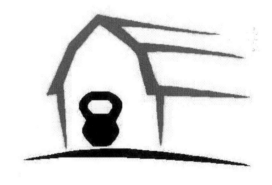

"THOSE WHO THINK THEY HAVE NOT TIME FOR BODILY EXERCISE WILL SOONER OR LATER HAVE TO FIND TIME FOR ILLNESS."

— EDWARD STANLEY

THE WORKOUTS

Workout 1:
(Perform 1-3 Rounds)
15 Push-ups followed by 15 Sit-ups
14 Push-ups followed by 14 Sit-ups
And so on...until you complete 1 Push-up followed by 1 Sit-up

Notes:

Workout 2:
(Perform for 20 Minutes)
10 Broad Jumps
30 Seconds of Bear Crawls
10 Broad Jumps
30 Seconds of Crab Walks

Notes:

Workout 3:
(Perform 8-10 Rounds)
30 Seconds of Mountain Climbers
15 Supermans
30 Seconds of Side-to-side Hops
15 Pull-ups

Notes:

Workout 4:

100 Lunges (each side)
15-Minute Run

Notes:

Workout 5:

Starting at minute 0, perform the exercise for 20 seconds, followed by 10 seconds of rest. At the 30-second mark, perform the same exercise another 20 seconds, followed by 10 seconds of rest. Repeat this process for a total of 8 times; therefore, you finish at the 4-minute mark. (This is known as Tabata.)

Tabata 1: Staggered Push-ups
(1-Minute Rest)
Tabata 2: Climbers
(1-Minute Rest)
Tabata 3: Wipers
(1-Minute Rest)
Tabata 4: Front Kicks

Notes:

Workout 6:

Starting at minute 0, perform the exercise for 10 seconds, followed by 10 seconds of rest. At the 20-second mark, perform the same exercise for 20 seconds, followed by 20 seconds of rest. Repeat this process, adding 10 seconds per round, until you can no longer perform the exercise.

Round 1:
10 Seconds of Wall Squat – Start 0:00, End 0:10
(10-Second Rest) – Start 0:10, End 0:20
20 Seconds of Wall Squat – Start 0:20, End 0:40
(20-Second Rest) – Start 0:40, End 1:00
And so on...

(2-Minute Rest, then...)
1 Minute of Uppercut Punches
1 Minute of Punches
1 Minute of Uppercut Punches
1 Minute of Punches
(Then...)

Round 2:
10 Seconds of Plank – Start 0:00, End 0:10
(10-Second Rest) – Start 0:10, End 0:20
20 Seconds of Plank – Start 0:20, End 0:40
(20-Second Rest) – Start 0:40, End 1:00
And so on...

Notes:

Workout 7:
(Perform 5-7 Rounds)
400-Meter Run
15 Burpees

Notes:

Workout 8:
Starting at minute 0, perform 10 Dips, followed by Single-leg Deadlifts for the remainder of the minute. At the beginning of the next minute (minute 1), once again perform 10 Dips followed by Single-leg Deadlifts for the remainder of the minute. Continue this process until you reach 100 Single-leg Deadlifts (each side).

Notes:

Workout 9:
(Perform 8-10 Rounds)
15 Pike Push-ups
20 Calf Raises
15 Sit-ups
20 Bridges

Notes:

Workout 10:
(Perform for 20 Minutes)
10 Pull-ups
30 Seconds of Dragon Walks
30 Jumping Jacks
30 Seconds of Plank Jumping Jacks

Notes:

Workout 11:
(Perform 3-5 Rounds)
3 Minutes of Bicycles
2 Minutes of Punches
(30-Second Rest)

Notes:

Workout 12:
(Perform for 20 Minutes)
30 Seconds of Butt Kicks
5 Diamond Push-ups
30 Seconds of Lunges
10 Wide Push-ups
30 Seconds of Deadlifts
5 Diamond Push-ups
30 Seconds of Air Squats
10 Wide Push-ups

Notes:

Workout 13:
(Perform 8-10 Rounds)
30 Seconds of Right-side Plank
30 Seconds of High Knees
30 Seconds of Left-side Plank
30 Seconds of Heismans

Notes:

Workout 14:
(Perform for 20 Minutes)
10 Pull-ups (Even Minutes – 0, 2, and so on...)
20 Leg Lifts (Odd Minutes – 1, 3, and so on...)

Notes:

Workout 15:
(Perform 5-7 Rounds)
2 Minutes of Jumping Jacks
1 Minute of Mountain Climbers
30 Seconds of Skaters

Notes:

Workout 16:
(Perform 8-10 Rounds)
25 Calf Raises
20 Toe Touches
15 Push-ups
10 Jump Squats

Notes:

Workout 17:
12 Inchworms followed by 12 Supermans
11 Inchworms followed by 11 Supermans
And so on...until you complete 1 Inchworm followed by 1 Superman

(Then...Perform 3-5 Rounds)
30 Seconds of Donkey Kicks
30 Seconds of Crab Kicks

Notes:

Workout 18:

5 Minutes of Burpees
(1-Minute Rest)
3 Minutes of Burpees
(1-Minute Rest)
1 Minute of Burpees
(1-Minute Rest)
5 Minutes of Burpees

Notes:

Workout 19:

Starting at minute 0, perform Skaters for 30 seconds, followed by rest for the remainder of the minute. At the beginning of the next minute (minute 1), perform as many Wipers as you can. Repeat this process until you reach 150 Wipers (side-to-side is 1).

Notes:

Workout 20:

Starting at minute 0, perform 15 Decline Push-ups, followed by rest for the remainder of the minute. At the beginning of the next minute (minute 1), perform as many Jump-overs as you can. Repeat this process until you reach 200 Jump-overs (front-to-back is 1).

Notes:

Workout 21:
(Perform 3-5 Rounds)
1 Minute of Foot-to-foot Crunches
800-Meter Run

Notes:

Workout 22:
(Perform 1-3 Rounds)
30 Seconds of Plank Jumps
30 Seconds of Toy Soldiers

(Then...)
15 Pike Push-ups followed by 1 Plank Reach (each side)
14 Pike Push-ups followed by 2 Plank Reaches (each side)
And so on...until you complete 1 Pike Push-up followed by
15 Plank Reaches (each side)

(Then...Perform 1-3 Rounds)
30 Seconds of Plank Jumps
30 Seconds of Toy Soldiers

Notes:

Workout 23:
1 Minute of Uppercut Punches
100 Deadlifts
1 Minute of Uppercut Punches
100 Air Squats
1 Minute of Uppercut Punches
50 Deadlifts
1 Minute of Uppercut Punches
50 Air Squats
1 Minute of Uppercut Punches

Notes:

Workout 24:
(Perform for 20 Minutes)
1 Chin-up followed by 1 Handstand Push-up
2 Chin-ups followed by 2 Handstand Push-ups
3 Chin-ups followed by 3 Handstand Push-ups
4 Chin-ups followed by 4 Handstand Push-ups
5 Chin-ups followed by 5 Handstand Push-ups

Notes:

Workout 25:
(Perform 3-5 Rounds)
30 Seconds of Right-side Plank Twists
1 Minute of Step-ups
1 Minute of Plank
1 Minute of Jump-overs
30 Seconds of Left-side Plank Twists

Notes:

Workout 26:
(Perform for 20 Minutes)
1 Minute of Inchworms
10 Jump Squats
1 Minute of Plank Jumps
10 Jump Squats

Notes:

Workout 27:
(Perform 5-7 Rounds)
30 Seconds of Crab Walks
1 Minute of Flutter Kicks
30 Seconds of Dragon Walks
1 Minute of Foot-to-foot Crunches

Notes:

Workout 28:
(Perform 1-3 Rounds)
5 Reverse Flyes followed by 10 Jumping Jacks
10 Reverse Flyes followed by 20 Jumping Jacks
15 Reverse Flyes followed by 30 Jumping Jacks
20 Reverse Flyes followed by 40 Jumping Jacks
25 Reverse Flyes followed by 50 Jumping Jacks
25 Reverse Flyes followed by 50 Jumping Jacks
20 Reverse Flyes followed by 40 Jumping Jacks
15 Reverse Flyes followed by 30 Jumping Jacks
10 Reverse Flyes followed by 20 Jumping Jacks
5 Reverse Flyes followed by 10 Jumping Jacks

Notes:

Workout 29:
Starting at minute 0, perform 15 Air Squats, followed by rest for the remainder of the minute. At the beginning of the next minute (minute 1), once again perform 15 Air Squats, again followed by rest for the remainder of the minute. Repeat this process until you have worked out for 20 Minutes (your final minute to perform Air Squats is minute 19).

Notes:

Workout 30:
(Perform 8-10 Rounds)
5 Handstand Push-ups
1 Minute of Heismans
10 Pike Push-ups
1 Minute of Toe Touches

Notes:

Workout 31:
(Perform for 20 Minutes)
10 Bridges
10 Jump-overs (front-to-back is 1)
10 Donkey Kicks (each side)
10 Step-ups

Notes:

Workout 32:
(Perform 8-10 Rounds)
200-Meter Run
20 Leg Lifts

Notes:

Workout 33:
(Perform 5-7 Rounds)
30 Seconds of Right-side Shuffles
1 Minute of Windmills
1 Minute of Reverse Flyes
30 Seconds of Left-side Shuffles

Notes:

Workout 34:
Starting at minute 0, perform the exercise for 20 seconds, followed by 10 seconds of rest. At the 30-second mark, perform the same exercise for another 20 seconds, followed by 10 seconds of rest. Repeat this process for a total of 8 times; therefore, you finish at the four-minute mark.

Tabata 1: Side-to-side Hops
(1-Minute Rest)
Tabata 2: Front Kicks
(1-Minute Rest)
Tabata 3: Burpee Push-ups
(1-Minute Rest)
Tabata 4: Burpee Sit-ups

Notes:

Workout 35:
Starting at minute 0, perform 30 Seconds of Wall Squat, followed by rest for the remainder of the minute. At the beginning of the next minute (minute 1), once again perform 30 Seconds of Wall Squat followed by rest for the remainder of the minute. Repeat this process until you have worked out for 20 Minutes.

Notes:

Workout 36:
(Perform for 20 Minutes)
5 Wall Walks
10 Sit-ups
15 Single-leg Deadlifts (each side)

Notes:

Workout 37:
(Perform for 20 Minutes)
10 Inchworm Push-ups
30 Seconds of High Knees
10 Hindu Push-ups
30 Seconds of Butt Kicks

Notes:

Workout 38:
(Perform 8-10 Rounds)
5 Burpee Broad Jumps
10 Dips
30 Seconds of Climbers

Notes:

Workout 39:
(Perform 1-3 Rounds)
10 Step-ups followed by 10 Staggered Push-ups
10 Step-ups followed by 10 Staggered Push-ups
And so on...until you complete 1 Step-up followed by 1 Staggered Push-up

Notes:

Workout 40:
(Perform 5-7 Rounds)
30 Seconds of Tuck Jumps
30 Seconds of Right-side Plank Twists
30 Seconds of Tuck Jumps
30 Seconds of Left-side Plank Twists
1 Minute of Bicycles

Notes:

Workout 41:
(Perform 3-5 Rounds)
1 Minute of Windmills
1 Minute of High Knees
1 Minute of Butt Kicks
50 Jumping Jacks

Notes:

Workout 42:
2 Minutes of Side-to-side Hops
100 Crunches
2 Minutes of Side-to-side Hops
75 Knee Lifts
2 Minutes of Side-to-side Hops
50 Crunches
2 Minutes of Side-to-side Hops
25 Knee Lifts
2 Minutes of Side-to-side Hops

Notes:

Workout 43:
(Perform 3-5 Rounds)
10 Lunges (each side)
1 Minute of Punches
1 Minute of Wall Squat
1 Minute of Uppercut Punches

Notes:

Workout 44:
(Perform for 20 Minutes)
50 Reverse Flyes
40 Sit-ups
30 Incline Push-ups
20 Supermans
10 Decline Push-ups

Notes:

Workout 45:
(Perform for 20 Minutes)
30 Seconds of Right-side Plank (Even Minutes – 0, 2, and so on...)
30 Seconds of Left-side Plank (Odd Minutes – 1, 3, and so on...)

Notes:

Workout 46:
Starting at minute 0, perform 1 Broad Jump, followed by 1 Plank Jumping Jack, followed by rest for the remainder of the minute. At the beginning of the next minute (minute 1), once again perform this process, but add 1 repetition to both exercises. Continue this process, adding 1 repetition to both exercises each round until you reach 20 repetitions of both the Broad Jump and Plank Jumping Jack, or until you can no longer perform the workout.

Notes:

Workout 47:
(Perform 5-7 Rounds)
7 Pull-ups
5 Jump Squats
14 Supermans
5 Jump Squats
21 Reverse Flyes
5 Jump Squats

Notes:

Workout 48:
(Perform 8-10 Rounds)
10 Burpees
1 Minute of Crunches

Notes:

Workout 49:
2 Minutes of Knee Lifts
100 Push-ups
100 Air Squats
2 Minutes of Knee Lifts
50 Lunges (each side)
50 Dips
2 Minutes of Knee Lifts

Notes:

Workout 50:
(Perform 8-10 Rounds)
30 Seconds of Right-side Shuffles
20 Windmills (side-to-side is 1)
20 Reverse Flyes
30 Seconds of Left-side Shuffles

Notes:

Workout 51:
(Perform for 20 Minutes)
30 Seconds of Climbers
5 Handstand Push-ups
30 Seconds of Heismans
5 Handstand Push-ups

Notes:

Workout 52:
(Perform 3-5 Rounds)
1 Minute of Front Kicks
1 Minute of Punches
1 Minute of Kickbacks
1 Minute of Uppercut Punches

Notes:

Workout 53:
(Perform 8-10 Rounds)
1 Minute of Mountain Climbers
1 Minute of Foot-to-foot Crunches

Notes:

Workout 54:
(Perform 3-5 Rounds)
1 Push-up followed by 1 Chin-up
2 Push-ups followed by 2 Chin-ups
3 Push-ups followed by 3 Chin-ups
4 Push-ups followed by 4 Chin-ups
5 Push-ups followed by 5 Chin-ups
4 Push-ups followed by 4 Chin-ups
3 Push-ups followed by 3 Chin-ups
2 Push-ups followed by 2 Chin-ups
1 Push-up followed by 1 Chin-up

Notes:

Workout 55:
(Perform 8-10 Rounds)
30 Seconds of Climbers
10 Burpee Broad Jumps
30 Seconds of Skaters

Notes:

Workout 56:
2 Minutes of Bear Crawls
20 Air Squats followed by 20 Plank Jumping Jacks
19 Air Squats followed by 19 Plank Jumping Jacks
And so on...until you complete 1 Air Squat followed by 1 Plank Jumping Jack
2 Minutes of Bear Crawls

Notes:

Workout 57:
Starting at minute 0, perform 5 Inchworm Push-ups, followed by rest for the remainder of the minute. At the beginning of the next minute (minute 1), perform 5 Inchworm Push-ups, again followed by rest for the remainder of the minute. Repeat this process until you reach 20 minutes of working out.

Notes:

Workout 58:
(Perform 5-7 Rounds)
1 Minute of Burpees
30 Seconds of Mountain Climbers
1 Minute of Side-to-side Hops
30 Seconds of Crab Kicks

Notes:

Workout 59:
2 Minutes of Dragon Walks
1 Minute of Bicycles
30 Seconds of Dragon Walks
50 Air Squats
40 Toe Touches
30 Jump Squats
20 Leg Lifts
10 Tuck Jumps
2 Minutes of Bicycles
1 Minute of Dragon Walks
30 Seconds of Bicycles

Notes:

Workout 60:
Starting at minute 0, perform 1 Diamond Push-up, followed by 1 Jump-over (front-to-back is 1), followed by rest for the remainder of the minute. At the beginning of the next minute (minute 1), once again perform this process, but add 1 repetition to both exercises. Continue this process, adding 1 repetition to both exercises each round until you reach 20 repetitions of both the Diamond Push-up and Jump-over, or until you can no longer perform the workout.

Notes:

Workout 61:
(Perform 1-3 Rounds)
1 Minute of Bridges
30 Reverse Flyes
1 Minute of Plank Reaches
25 Supermans
1 Minute of Butt Kicks
20 Reverse Flyes
1 Minute of Bridges
15 Supermans
1 Minute of Plank Reaches
10 Reverse Flyes
1 Minute of Butt Kicks
5 Supermans

Notes:

Workout 62:
(Perform 8-10 Rounds)
1 Minute of Flutter Kicks
1 Minute of Plank Jumps
20 Calf Raises

Notes:

Workout 63:
(Perform 8-10 Rounds)
30 Seconds of Bear Crawls
30 Seconds of Punches
30 Seconds of Crab Walks
30 Seconds of Heismans

Notes:

Workout 64:
(Perform 5-7 Rounds)
15 Jump Squats
20 Staggered Push-ups
15 Tuck Jumps
20 Wipers (side-to-side is 1)

Notes:

Workout 65:
(Perform 5-7 Rounds)
30 Seconds of Right-side Plank Twists
30 Seconds of Front Kicks
1 Minute of Plank
30 Seconds of Kickbacks
30 Seconds of Left-side Plank Twists

Notes:

Workout 66:
(Perform 8-10 Rounds)
5 Handstand Push-ups
10 Pull-ups
20 Deadlifts

Notes:

Workout 67:
100 Inchworm Push-ups or Inchworm Push-ups for 20 minutes, whichever comes first.

Notes:

Workout 68:
1 Minute of Sit-ups
5-Minute Run
1 Minute of Sit-ups
4-Minute Run
1 Minute of Sit-ups
3-Minute Run
1 Minute of Sit-ups
2-Minute Run
1 Minute of Sit-ups
1-Minute Run
1 Minute of Sit-ups

Notes:

Workout 69:
(Perform 3-5 Rounds)
1 Minute of Punches
3 Air Squats followed by 1 Dip
6 Air Squats followed by 2 Dips
9 Air Squats followed by 3 Dips
12 Air Squats followed by 4 Dips
15 Air Squats followed by 5 Dips
1 Minute of Uppercut Punches

Notes:

Workout 70:
Starting at minute 0, perform the exercise for 10 seconds, followed by 10 seconds of rest. At the 20-second mark, perform the same exercise for 20 seconds, followed by 20 seconds of rest. Continue this process, adding 10 seconds per round, until you reach 20 minutes of one exercise or until you can no longer perform the exercise.

Round 1:
10 Seconds of Frozen V Sit – Start 0:00, End 0:10
(10-Second Rest) – Start 0:10, End 0:20
20 Seconds of Frozen V Sit – Start 0:20, End 0:40
(20-Second Rest) – Start 0:40, End 1:00
And so on...

(2-Minute Rest)

Round 2:
10 Seconds of Jumping Jack Planks – Start 0:00, End 0:10
(10-Second Rest) – Start 0:10, End 0:20
20 Seconds of Jumping Jack Planks – Start 0:20, End 0:40
(20-Second Rest) – Start 0:40, End 1:00
And so on...

Notes:

Workout 71:
(Perform 8-10 Rounds)
10 Broad Jumps
30 Seconds of Crab Walks
30 Seconds of Toy Soldiers
30 Seconds of Crab Kicks

Notes:

Workout 72:
(Perform for 20 Minutes)
1 Minute of Flutter Kicks
15 Decline Push-ups
1 Minute of Leg Lifts
15 Incline Push-ups

Notes:

Workout 73:
12 Lunges (each side) followed by 1 Windmill (side-to-side is 1)
11 Lunges (each side) followed by 2 Windmills (side-to-side is 1)
And so on...until you complete 1 Lunge (each side) followed by 12 Windmills (side-to-side is 1)

(Then...Perform 1-3 Rounds)
2 Minutes of High Knees
1 Minute of Deadlifts
30 Seconds of Air Squats

Notes:

Workout 74:
(Perform 3-5 Rounds)
1 Minute of Mountain Climbers
15 Calf Raises
30 Seconds of Right-side Plank
30 Seconds of Left-side Plank
15 Calf Raises
1 Minute of Kickbacks

Notes:

Workout 75:
(Perform for 20 Minutes)
10 Pike Push-ups
30 Seconds of Right-side Shuffles
5 Superman Push-ups
30 Seconds of Left-side Shuffles

Notes:

Workout 76:
Starting at minute 0, perform the exercise for 20 seconds, followed by 10 seconds of rest. At the 30-second mark, perform the same exercise another 20 seconds, followed by 10 seconds of rest. Repeat this process for a total of 8 times; therefore, you finish at the four-minute mark.

Tabata 1: Heismans
(1-Minute Rest)
Tabata 2: Punches
(1-Minute Rest)
Tabata 3: Toy Soldiers
(1-Minute Rest)
Tabata 4: Crunches

Notes:

Workout 77:
(Perform for 20 Minutes)
30 Seconds of Dragon Walks
3 Bridges
6 Jump Squats
9 Donkey Kicks (each side)
12 Lunges (each side)

Notes:

Workout 78:
(Perform 8-10 Rounds)
30 Seconds of Skaters
1 Minute of Jumping Jacks
20 Incline Push-ups

Notes:

Workout 79:
(Perform for 20 Minutes)
400-Meter Run
20 Sit-ups

Notes:

Workout 80:
(Perform 8-10 Rounds)
30 Seconds of Dragon Walks
30 Seconds of Broad Jumps
30 Seconds of Butt Kicks
30 Seconds of Plank Jumps

Notes:

Workout 81:
4 Minutes of Burpee Push-ups
(2-Minute Rest)
4 Minutes of Burpee Push-ups
(2-Minute Rest)
4 Minutes of Burpee Push-ups

Notes:

Workout 82:
(Perform for 20 Minutes)
7 Inchworms (Even Minutes – 0, 2, and so on…)
20 Bridges (Odd Minutes – 1, 3, and so on…)

Notes:

Workout 83:
(Perform 3-5 Rounds)
30 Seconds of High Knees
30 Seconds of Right-side Plank
30 Seconds of Kickbacks
30 Sit-ups
30 Seconds of High Knees
30 Seconds of Left-side Plank
30 Seconds of Kickbacks
30 Leg Lifts

Notes:

Workout 84:
(Perform 3-5 Rounds)
1 Minute of Side-to-side Hops
15 Decline Push-ups
1 Minute of Side-to-side Hops
15 Dips
1 Minute of Side-to-side Hops
15 Incline Push-ups

Notes:

Workout 85:
(Perform for 20 Minutes)
10 Chin-ups
30 Seconds of Right-side Shuffles
20 Toe Touches
30 Seconds of Left-side Shuffles

Notes:

Workout 86:
Starting at minute 0, perform 3 Handstand Push-ups, followed by as many Reverse Flyes as you can for the remainder of the minute. At the beginning of the next minute (minute 1), once again perform 3 Handstand Push-ups, followed by as many Reverse Flyes as you can for the remainder of the minute. Repeat this process until you reach 200 Reverse Flyes.

Notes:

Workout 87:
Starting at minute 0, perform Bear Crawls for the entire minute. At the beginning of the next minute (minute 1), perform Step-ups for the entire minute. Repeat this process until you reach 150 Step-ups.

Notes:

Workout 88:
(Perform for 20 Minutes)
5 Dips
10 Bridges
15 Push-ups
20 Wipers (side-to-side is 1)

Notes:

Workout 89:
(Perform 3-5 Rounds)
5-Minute Run
1 Minute of Plank

Notes:

Workout 90:
(Perform for 20 Minutes)
3 Pull-ups
6 Burpees
9 Jumping Jacks
12 Donkey Kicks (each side)

Notes:

Workout 91:
(Perform 5-7 Rounds)
30 Seconds of Right-side Plank Twists
1 Minute of Climbers
30 Seconds of Plank Jumping Jacks
1 Minute of Butt Kicks
30 Seconds of Left-side Plank Twists

Notes:

Workout 92:
Round 1:
Perform 100 Lunges (each side)

(2-Minute Rest)

Round 2:
Starting at minute 0, perform Wall Squats for 10 seconds, followed by 10 seconds of rest. At the 20-second mark, perform Wall Squats for 20 seconds, followed by 20 seconds of rest. Continue this process, adding 10 seconds per round, until you can no longer perform the exercise.

10 Seconds of Wall Squat – Start 0:00, End 0:10
(10-Second Rest) – Start 0:10, End 0:20
20 Seconds of Wall Squat – Start 0:20, End 0:40
(20-Second Rest) – Start 0:40, End 1:00
And so on...

Notes:

Workout 93:
(Perform for 20 Minutes)
10 Staggered Push-ups (Even Minutes – 0, 2, and so on...)
5 Burpee Sit-ups (Odd Minutes – 1, 3, and so on...)

Notes:

Workout 94:
15 Wipers (side-to-side is 1) followed by 1 Bridge
14 Wipers (side-to-side is 1) followed by 2 Bridges
And so on... until you complete 1 Wiper (side-to-side is 1)
followed by 15 Bridges

(Then...Perform 1-3 Rounds)
30 Deadlifts
20 Knee Lifts
10 Single-leg Deadlifts (each leg)
30 Seconds of Wipers
30 Seconds of Bridges

Notes:

Workout 95:
(Perform 3-5 Rounds)
15 Supermans
800-Meter Run
30 Toy Soldiers (each side)

Notes:

Workouts 96:
(Perform for 20 Minutes)
10 Pike Push-ups
20 Jump-overs (front-to-back is 1)
30 Air Squats

Notes:

Workout 97:
(Perform for 20 Minutes)
10 Diamond Push-ups
30 Seconds of Frozen V Sit
10 Dips
30 Seconds of Plank

Notes:

Workout 98:
Starting at minute 0, perform the exercise for 20 seconds, followed by 10 seconds of rest. At the 30-second mark, perform the same exercise another 20 seconds, followed by 10 seconds of rest. Repeat this process a total of 8 times; therefore, you finish at the four-minute mark.

Tabata 1: Deadlifts
(1-Minute Rest)
Tabata 2: Flutter Kicks
(1-Minute Rest)
Tabata 3: Windmills
(1-Minute Rest)
Tabata 4: Plank Reaches

Notes:

Workout 99:
(Perform 1-3 Rounds)
15 Jumping Jacks followed by 15 Plank Jumping Jacks
14 Jumping Jacks followed by 14 Plank Jumping Jacks
And so on...until you complete 1 Jumping Jack followed by 1 Plank Jumping Jack

Notes:

Workout 100:
(Perform 5-7 Rounds)
30 Seconds of Uppercut Punches
5 Superman Push-ups
30 Seconds of Right-side Plank
5 Superman Push-ups
30 Seconds of Left-side Plank
5 Superman Push-ups
30 Seconds of Punches
5 Superman Push-ups

Notes:

Workout 101:
(Perform 8-10 Rounds)
30 Seconds of Tuck Jumps
30 Seconds of Bear Crawl

(1-Minute Rest, then...)
50 Burpee Broad Jumps

Notes:

Workout 102:
(Perform for 20 Minutes)
30 Seconds of Crab Walks
30 Seconds of Dragon Walks
10 Chin-ups

Notes:

Workout 103:
Starting at minute 0, perform 1 Inchworm Push-up, followed by 1 Knee Lift, followed by rest for the remainder of the minute. At the beginning of the next minute (minute 1), once again perform this process, but add 1 repetition to both exercises. Continue this process, adding 1 repetition to both exercises each round until you reach 20 repetitions of both the Inchworm Push-up and Knee Lift, or until you can no longer perform the workout.

Notes:

Workout 104:
(Perform 5-7 Rounds)
30 Seconds of Heismans
1 Minute of Side-to-side Hops
30 Seconds of Plank Jumps
1 Minute of Punches

Notes:

Workout 105:
(Perform for 20 Minutes)
5 Pull-ups
10 Jump Squats
15 Sit-ups

Notes:

Workout 106:
(Perform 1-3 Rounds)
1-Mile Run
(2-Minute Rest)

Notes:

Workout 107:
(Perform for 20 Minutes)
5 Diamond Push-ups
5 Leg Lifts
5 Wide Push-ups
5 Knee Lifts
5 Superman Push-ups
5 Toe Touches

Notes:

Workout 108:
(Perform for 20 Minutes)
40 Deadlifts
20 Burpees
10 Tuck Jumps

Notes:

Workout 109:
(Perform 8-10 Rounds)
20 Supermans
20 Crunches
1 Minute of Reverse Flyes
1 Minute of Flutter Kicks

Notes:

Workout 110:
Starting at minute 0, perform 3 Handstand Push-ups, followed by Push-ups for the remainder of the minute. At the beginning of the next minute (minute 1), once again perform 3 Handstand Push-ups, followed by Push-ups for the remainder of the minute. Continue this process until you reach 125 Push-ups.

Notes:

Workout 111:

Starting at minute 0, perform 10 Windmills (side-to-side is 1), followed by Air Squats for the remainder of the minute. At the beginning of the next minute (minute 1), once again perform 10 Windmills (side-to-side is 1), followed by Air Squats for the remainder of the minute. Repeat this process until you reach 150 Air Squats.

Notes:

Workout 112:

(Perform 5-7 Rounds)
10 Pull-ups
1 Minute of High Knees
10 Chin-ups
1 Minute of Jump-overs

Notes:

Workout 113:

(Perform 5-7 Rounds)
30 Seconds of Right-side Shuffles
10 Burpee Sit-ups
30 Seconds of Left-side Shuffles
10 Burpee Sit-ups

Notes:

Workout 114:
(Perform for 20 Minutes)
10 Hindu Push-ups (Even Minutes – 0, 2, and so on…)
5 Inchworms (Odd Minutes – 1, 3, and so on…)

Notes:

Workout 115:
(Perform 3-5 Rounds)
800-Meter Run
20 Air Squats
10 Leg Lifts

Notes:

Workout 116:
(Perform 8-10 Rounds)
5 Burpees
10 Dips
15 Supermans
20 Calf Raises

Notes:

Workout 117:
(Perform 1-3 Rounds)
50 Butt Kicks (each side)
50 Jumping Jacks
50 Climbers (each side)
50 Side-to-side Hops (side-to-side is 1)
50 High Knees (each side)
50 Jump-overs (front-to-back is 1)

Notes:

Workout 118:
(Perform 8-10 Rounds)
30 Seconds of Mountain Climbers
30 Seconds of Punches
30 Seconds of Donkey Kicks
30 Seconds of Uppercut Punches
30 Seconds of Plank

Notes:

Workout 119:
2 Minutes of Wall Walks

(Then...Perform 5-7 Rounds)
30 Seconds of Right-side Shuffles
10 Pike Push-ups
30 Seconds of Left-side Shuffles
5 Pike Push-ups

Notes:

Workout 120:
(Perform for 20 Minutes)
30 Seconds of Dragon Walks
20 Lunges (each side)
20 Leg Lifts

Notes:

Workout 121:
Starting at minute 0, perform 1 Pull-up, followed by 1 Dip, followed by rest for the remainder of the minute. At the beginning of the next minute (minute 1), once again perform this process, but add 1 repetition to the respective exercises. Continue this process, adding 1 repetition to both exercises each round until you reach 20 repetitions of Pull-up and Dip, or until you can no longer perform the workout.

Notes:

Workout 122:
10-Minute Run
5 Minutes of Crunches
10-Minute Run

Notes:

Workout 123:
4 Minutes of Burpee Broad Jumps
(1-Minute Rest)
3 Minutes of Burpee Broad Jumps
(1-Minute Rest)
2 Minutes of Burpee Broad Jumps
(1-Minute Rest)
1 Minute of Burpee Broad Jumps
(1-Minute Rest)
4 Minutes of Burpee Broad Jumps

Notes:

Workouts 124:
(Perform for 20 Minutes)
10 Single-leg Deadlifts (each side)
10 Sit-ups
10 Chin-ups
10 Jumping Jacks

Notes:

Workout 125:
(Perform 8-10 Rounds)
30 Seconds of Crab Walks
30 Seconds of Front Kicks
30 Seconds of Kickbacks
30 Seconds of Bear Crawls
Notes:

Workout 126:
(Perform for 20 Minutes)
5 Diamond Push-ups (Even Minutes – 0, 2, and so on...)
10 Wide Push-ups (Odd Minutes – 1, 3, and so on...)

Notes:

Workout 127:
(Perform for 20 Minutes)
3 Burpee Push-ups
6 Air Squats
9 Burpee Push-ups
12 Air Squats

Notes:

Workout 128:
(Perform 8-10 Rounds)
1 Minute of Kickbacks
30 Seconds of Pike Push-ups
5 Sit-ups
10 Leg Lifts
15 Crunches

Notes:

Workout 129:
(Perform 5-7 Rounds)
30 Seconds of Toy Soldiers
30 Seconds of Tuck Jumps
30 Seconds of Heismans
30 Seconds of Deadlifts
30 Seconds of Calf Raises
30 Seconds of High Knees

Notes:

Workout 130:
(Perform 5-7 Rounds)
50 Reverse Flyes
30 Seconds of Plank Reaches
30 Seconds of Crab Kicks
30 Seconds of Punches

Notes:

Workout 131:
(Perform 8-10 Rounds)
10 Lunges (each side)
30 Seconds of Jumping Jacks
1 Minute of Bicycles

Notes:

Workout 132:
Starting at minute 0, perform 1 Burpee, followed by rest for the remainder of the minute. At the beginning of the next minute (minute 1), add 1 repetition to the exercise, and rest for the remainder of the minute. Continue this process, adding 1 repetition to the exercise each round until you reach 20 repetitions of the Burpee, or until you can no longer perform the exercise.

Notes:

Workout 133:
(Perform 5-7 Rounds)
1 Minute of Kickbacks
30 Seconds of Right-side Plank Twists
30 Seconds of Left-side Plank Twists
1 Minute of Front kicks

Notes:

Workout 134:
(Perform 1-3 Rounds)
50 Jumping Jacks
40 Bridges
30 Supermans
20 Crunches
10 Burpee Sit-ups

Notes:

Workout 135:
(Perform for 20 Minutes)
20 Dips
20 Deadlifts
20 Hindu Push-ups
20 Butt Kicks (each side)

Notes:

Workout 136:
(Perform for 20 Minutes)
5 Handstand Push-ups
10 Tuck Jumps
15 Pike Push-ups
20 Air Squats

Notes:

Workout 137:
(Perform 5-7 Rounds)
1 Minute of Inchworms
15 Pull-ups
1 Minute of Climbers
20 Wipers (side-to-side is 1)

Notes:

Workout 138:
(Perform for 20 Minutes)
5 Superman Push-ups
10 Supermans
15 Decline Push-ups
20 Reverse Flyes
25 Incline Push-ups
30 Seconds of Crab Kicks

Notes:

Workout 139:
(Perform for 20 Minutes)
30 Seconds of Lunges
10 Inchworms
30 Seconds of Donkey Kicks

Notes:

Workout 140:
(Perform 8-10 Rounds)
30 Seconds of Front Kicks
30 Seconds of Plank Jumping Jacks
30 Seconds of Toy Soldiers
30 Seconds of Plank

Notes:

Workout 141:
Starting at minute 0, perform 1 Toe Touch, followed by 1 Windmill (side-to-side is 1), followed by rest for the remainder of the minute. At the beginning of the next minute (minute 1), once again perform this process, but add 1 repetition to both exercises. Continue this process, adding 1 repetition to both exercises each round until you reach 20 repetitions of both the Toe Touch and Windmill, or until you can no longer perform the workout.

Notes:

Workout 142:

1-Mile Run
10 Air Squats
800-Meter Run
20 Air Squats
400-Meter Run
30 Air Squats
200-Meter Run
40 Air Squats

Notes:

Workout 143:

(Perform 3-5 Rounds)
1 Minute of Mountain Climbers
1 Minute of Punches
1 Minute of Plank Jumps
1 Minute of Punches

Notes:

Workout 144:
(Perform for 20 Minutes)
30 Seconds of Butt Kicks
10 Decline Push-ups
30 Seconds of High Knees
10 Hindu Push-ups

Notes:

Workout 145:
(Perform 1-3 Rounds)
1 Minute of Plank
1 Minute of Wipers
1 Minute of Flutter Kicks
1 Minute of Sit-ups
(1-Minute Rest)
1 Minute of Plank Reaches
1 Minute of Knee Lifts
1 Minute of Crunches
1 Minute of Toe Touches
(1-Minute Rest)

Notes:

Workout 146:
400-Meter Run

(Then...)
Starting at minute 0, perform 5 Pike Push-ups, followed by Jumping Jacks for the remainder of the minute. At the beginning of the next minute (minute 1), once again perform 5 Pike Push-ups, followed by Jumping Jacks for the remainder of the minute. Repeat this process until you reach 200 Jumping Jacks.

(Then...)
400-Meter Run

Notes:

Workout 147:
(Perform for 8-10 Rounds)
30 Seconds of Climbers
30 Seconds of Donkey Kicks
30 Seconds of Crab Kicks
30 Seconds of Wall Squat

Notes:

Workout 148:
(Perform for 20 Minutes)
12 Chin-ups followed by 1 Dip
11 Chin-ups followed by 2 Dips
And so on…until you complete 1 Chin-up followed by 12 Dips

Notes:

Workout 149:
(Perform 3-5 Rounds)
4-Minute Run
1 Minute of Foot-to-foot Crunches
30 Seconds of Knee Lifts

Notes:

Workout 150:
Starting at minute 0, perform the exercise for 10 seconds, followed by 10 seconds of rest. At the 20-second mark, perform the same exercise for 20 seconds, followed by 20 seconds of rest. Continue this process, adding 10 seconds per round, until you can no longer perform the exercise.

Round 1:
10 Seconds of Right-side Plank – Start 0:00, End 0:10
(10-Second Rest) – Start 0:10, End 0:20
20 Seconds of Right-side Plank – Start 0:20, End 0:40
(20-Second Rest) – Start 0:40, End 1:00
And so on…

(2-Minute Rest)

Round 2:
10 Seconds of Left-side Plank – Start 0:00, End 0:10
(10-Second Rest) – Start 0:10, End 0:20
20 Seconds of Left-side Plank – Start 0:20, End 0:40
(20-Second Rest) – Start 0:40, End 1:00
And so on...

(2-Minute Rest)

Round 3:
10 Seconds of Plank – Start 0:00, End 0:10
(10-Second Rest) – Start 0:10, End 0:20
20 Seconds of Plank – Start 0:20, End 0:40
(20-Second Rest) – Start 0:40, End 1:00
And so on...

Notes:

Workout 151:
(Perform 5-7 Rounds)
30 Seconds of Dragon Walks
1 Minute of Side-to-side Hops
30 Seconds of Bear Crawls
1 Minute of Jump-overs

Notes:

Workout 152:
(Perform for 20 Minutes)
5 Push-ups
10 Sit-ups
15 Air Squats

Notes:

Workout 153:
(Perform for 20 Minutes)
20 Windmills (side-to-side is 1)
10 Chin-ups
15 Deadlifts
5 Pull-ups

Notes:

Workout 154:
Starting at minute 0, perform 1 Pike Push-up, followed by 1 Calf Raise, followed by rest for the remainder of the minute. At the beginning of the next minute (minute 1), once again perform this process, but add 1 repetition to both exercises. Continue this process, adding 1 repetition to both exercises each round until you reach 20 repetitions of both the Pike Push-up and Calf Raise, or until you can no longer perform the workout.

Notes:

Workout 155:
(Perform for 20 Minutes)
30 Seconds of Right-side Plank Twists
10 Burpee Sit-ups
20 Supermans
10 Burpee Sit-ups
30 Seconds of Left-side Plank Twists

Notes:

Workout 156:
(Perform 3-5 Rounds)
30 Seconds of Deadlifts
1 Dip followed by 1 Plank Jumping Jack
2 Dips followed by 2 Plank Jumping Jacks
3 Dips followed by 3 Plank Jumping Jacks
4 Dips followed by 4 Plank Jumping Jacks
5 Dips followed by 5 Plank Jumping Jacks
4 Dips followed by 4 Plank Jumping Jacks
3 Dips followed by 3 Plank Jumping Jacks
2 Dips followed by 2 Plank Jumping Jacks
1 Dip followed by 1 Plank Jumping Jack
30 Seconds of Toy Soldiers

Notes:

Workout 157:
(Perform 5-7 Rounds)
30 Jumping Jacks
1 Minute of Wall Squat
1 Minute of Jump-overs
15 Burpees

Notes:

Workout 158:
(Perform 3-5 Rounds)
1 Minute of Skaters
1 Minute of Punches
1 Minute of Step-ups
1 Minute of Uppercut Punches

Notes:

Workout 159:
Perform as many Staggered Push-ups as you can, followed by Tuck Jumps until you near fatigue. Start again performing as many Staggered Push-ups as you can, then as many Tuck Jumps as you can. Continue this process until you reach 100 Staggered Push-ups and 100 Tuck Jumps.

(Then...)
1-Mile Run

Notes:

Workout 160:
(Perform 3-5 Rounds)
2 Wall Walks
4 Sit-ups
6 Pike Push-ups
8 Donkey Kicks (each side)
10 Leg Lifts
8 Donkey Kicks (each side)
6 Pike Push-ups
4 Sit-ups
2 Wall Walks

Notes:

Workout 161:
(Perform for 20 Minutes)
20 Jump Squats
20 Supermans
20 Calf Raises
30 Seconds of Crab Kicks

Notes:

Workout 162:
Starting at minute 0, perform 30 seconds of Flutter Kicks, followed by rest for the remainder of the minute. At the beginning of the next minute (minute 1), once again perform 30 seconds of Flutter Kicks, again followed by rest for the remainder of the minute. Repeat this process until you have worked out for 20 minutes.

Notes:

Workout 163:
(Perform for 20 Minutes)
15 Seconds of Inchworm Push-ups
15 Seconds of Calf Raises
15 Seconds of Hindu Push-ups
(30-Second Rest)

Notes:

Workout 164:
(Perform for 20 Minutes)
30 Seconds of Plank Jumping Jacks
1 Minute of Side-to-side Hops

Notes:

Workout 165:
Starting at minute 0, perform 3 Wall Walks, followed by Broad Jumps for the remainder of the minute. At the beginning of the next minute (minute 1), once again perform 3 Wall Walks, followed by Broad Jumps for the remainder of the minute. Repeat this process until you reach 125 Broad Jumps.

Notes:

Workout 166:
(Perform 8-10 Rounds)
20 Reverse Flyes
30 Seconds of Dragon Walks
10 Burpee Push-ups

Notes:

Workout 167:
Starting at minute 0, perform 1 Deadlift, followed by 1 Sit-up, followed by rest for the remainder of the minute. At the beginning of the next minute (minute 1), once again perform this process, but add 1 repetition to both exercises.
Continue this process, adding 1 repetition to both exercises each round until you reach 20 repetitions of both the Deadlift and Sit-up, or until you can no longer perform the workout.

Notes:

Workout 168:
(Perform 5-7 Rounds)
1 Minute of Bicycles
30 Seconds of Tuck Jumps
1 Minute of Plank Reaches
30 Seconds of Crab Kicks

Notes:

Workout 169:
(Perform for 20 Minutes)
15 Jump-overs (front-to-back is 1) followed by 30 Seconds of Mountain Climbers
14 Jump-overs (front-to-back is 1) followed by 30 Seconds of Mountain Climbers
And so on...until you complete 1 Jump-over (front-to-back is 1) followed by 30 Seconds of Mountain Climbers

Notes:

Workout 170:
(Perform 3-5 Rounds)
30 Seconds of Plank
4-Minute Run
30 Seconds of Knee Lifts

Notes:

Workout 171:
(Perform 5-7 Rounds)
30 Seconds of Punches
1 Burpee
30 Seconds of Uppercut Punches
2 Burpees
30 Seconds of Punches
3 Burpees
30 Seconds of Uppercut Punches
4 Burpees
30 Seconds of Punches
5 Burpees
30 Seconds of Uppercut Punches

Notes:

Workout 172:
Starting at minute 0, perform an exercise for 20 seconds, followed by 10 seconds of rest. At the 30-second mark, perform the same exercise another 20 seconds, followed by 10 seconds of rest. Repeat this process a total of 8 times; therefore, you finish at the 4-minute mark.

Tabata 1: Inchworms
(1-Minute Rest)
Tabata 2: Bear Crawls
(1-Minute Rest)
Tabata 3: Dragon Walks
(1-Minute Rest)
Tabata 4: Mountain Climbers

Notes:

Workout 173:
(Perform 8-10 Rounds)
30 Seconds of Lunges
30 Seconds of Push-ups
1 Minute of Jumping Jacks

Notes:

Workout 174:
(Perform for 20 Minutes)
20 Reverse Flyes
15 Bridges
10 Toe Touches
5 Inchworms

Notes:

Workout 175:
(Perform 3-5 Rounds)
20 Calf Raises
20 Pike Push-ups
20 Front Kicks (each side)
20 Windmills (side-to-side is 1)

Notes:

Workout 176:
Starting at minute 0, perform an exercise for 20 seconds, followed by 10 seconds of rest. At the 30-second mark, perform the same exercise another 20 seconds, followed by 10 seconds of rest. Repeat this process a total of 8 times; therefore, you finish at the four-minute mark.

Tabata 1: Lunges
(1-Minute Rest)
Tabata 2: Sit-ups
(1-Minute Rest)
Tabata 3: Air Squats
(1-Minute Rest)
Tabata 4: Bicycles

Notes:

Workout 177:
(Perform for 20 Minutes)
10 Decline Push-ups (Even Minutes – 0, 2, and so on…)
15 Seconds of Right-side Plank Twists followed by 15 Seconds of Left-side Plank Twists (Odd Minutes – 1, 3, and so on…)

Notes:

Workout 178:
(Perform for 20 Minutes)
15 Seconds of Heismans
15 Seconds of Climbers
15 Seconds of Kickbacks
(15-Second Rest)

Notes:

Workout 179:
(Perform 3-5 Rounds)
4-Minute Run
1 Minute of Air Squats

Notes:

Workout 180:
(Perform for 20 Minutes)
5 Diamond Push-ups
30 Seconds of High Knees
10 Push-ups
30 Seconds of Butt Kicks
15 Wide Push-ups
30 Seconds of Toy Soldiers

Notes:

Workout 181:
(Perform 5-7 Rounds)
30 Seconds of Dragon Walks
1 Minute of Donkey Kicks
30 Seconds of Frozen V Sit
1 Minute of Burpees

Notes:

Workout 182:
(Perform 8-10 Rounds)
30 Seconds of Bear Crawls
30 Seconds of Reverse Flyes
10 Pull-ups
30 Seconds of Skaters

Notes:

Workout 183:
Starting at minute 0, perform 30 Seconds of Crunches, followed by Wide Push-ups for the remainder of the minute. At the beginning of the next minute (minute 1), once again perform 30 Seconds of Crunches followed by Wide Push-ups for the remainder of the minute. Continue this process until you reach 125 Wide Push-ups.

Notes:

Workout 184:

Starting at minute 0, perform 3 Wall Walks, followed by Bridges for the remainder of the minute. At the beginning of the next minute (minute 1), once again perform 3 Wall Walks, followed by Bridges for the remainder of the minute. Repeat this process until you reach 125 Bridges.

Notes:

Workout 185:

(Perform 5-7 Rounds)
400-Meter Run
10 Burpee Sit-ups
10 Burpee Push-ups

Notes:

Workout 186:

1 Minute of Push-ups
2 Minutes of Bicycles

(Then...Perform 3-5 Rounds)
25 Incline Push-ups
2 Minutes of Side-to-side Hops
50 Knee Lifts
2 Minutes of Side-to-side Hops

Notes:

Workout 187:
(Perform 20 Rounds)
45 Seconds of Step-ups
(15-Second Rest)

Notes:

Workout 188:
Starting at minute 0, perform an exercise for 20 seconds, followed by 10 seconds of rest. At the 30-second mark, perform the same exercise another 20 seconds, followed by 10 seconds of rest. Repeat this process a total of 8 times; therefore, you finish at the four-minute mark.

Tabata 1: Inchworm Push-ups
(1-Minute Rest)
Tabata 2: Single-leg Deadlifts
(1-Minute Rest)
Tabata 3: Plank Jumping Jacks
(1-Minute Rest)
Tabata 4: Kickbacks

Notes:

Workout 189:
(Perform 8-10 Rounds)
30 Seconds of Left-side Shuffles
30 Seconds of Right-side Plank
30 Seconds of Left-side Plank
30 Seconds of Right-side Shuffles

Notes:

Workout 190:
(Perform 8-10 Rounds)
20 Bridges
30 Seconds of Crab Kicks
1 Minute of Plank Jumps

Notes:

Workout 191:
(Perform for 20 Minutes)
15 Air Squats
10 Push-ups
5 Burpee Sit-ups

Notes:

Workout 192:
2 Minutes of Plank
20-Minute Run
2 Minutes of Plank

Notes:

Workout 193:
(Perform 5-7 Rounds)
1 Minute of Jump-overs
10 Pull-ups
1 Minute of Side-to-side Hops
10 Pull-ups
1 Minute of Jumping Jacks
10 Pull-ups

Notes:

Workout 194:
(Perform 8-10 Rounds)
10 Pike Push-ups
30 Seconds of Right-side Shuffles
30 Seconds of Punches
30 Seconds of Left-side Shuffles

Notes:

Workout 195:
(Perform 3-5 Rounds)
30 Seconds of Bear Crawls
10 Burpee Broad Jumps
2 Minutes of Flutter Kicks
10 Tuck Jumps
30 Seconds of Calf Raises

Notes:

Workout 196:
(Perform 5-7 Rounds)
20 Single-leg Deadlifts (each side)
20 Reverse Flyes
20 Deadlifts
20 Chin-ups

Notes:

Workout 197:
(Perform 5-7 Rounds)
30 Seconds of Foot-to-foot Crunches
30 Seconds of Mountain Climbers
30 Seconds of Foot-to-foot Crunches
30 Seconds of Plank Jumps
30 Seconds of Foot-to-foot Crunches
30 Seconds of Plank Jumping Jacks
(30-Second Rest)

Notes:

Workout 198:
100 Push-ups
100 Sit-ups
100 Air Squats

Notes:

Workout 199:
(Perform 1-3 Rounds)
12 Tuck Jumps followed by 12 Plank Reaches (each side)
11 Tuck Jumps followed by 11 Plank Reaches (each side)
And so on...until you complete 1 Tuck Jump followed by 1 Plank Reach (each side)
30 Seconds of Crab Kicks
30 Seconds of Plank
30 Seconds of Crab Walk

Notes:

Workout 200:
(Perform for 3-5 Rounds)
3 Minutes of Jumping Jacks
2 Minutes of Toy Soldiers
1 Minute of Mountain Climbers
(1-Minute Rest)

Notes:

Workout 201:
(Perform for 20 Minutes)
20 Staggered Push-ups
25 Calf Raises
30 Leg Lifts

Notes:

Workout 202:
10 Burpees followed by 30 Seconds of Frozen V Sit
9 Burpees followed by 30 Seconds of Frozen V Sit
And so on...until you complete 1 Burpee followed by 30 Seconds of Frozen V Sit

Notes:

Workout 203:
(Perform 3-5 Rounds)
30 Seconds of Right-side Plank
30 Seconds of Dragon Walk
30 Seconds of Plank
30 Seconds of Tuck Jumps
30 Seconds of Left-side Plank
30 Seconds of Toy Soldiers

Notes:

Workout 204:
(Perform 3-5 Rounds)
5-Minute Run
1 Minute of Punches
1 Minute of Uppercut Punches

Notes:

Workout 205:
Starting at minute 0, perform 1 Jump Squat, followed by 1 Superman followed by rest for the remainder of the minute. At the beginning of the next minute (minute 1), once again perform this process, but add 1 repetition to both exercises. Continue this process, adding 1 repetition to both exercises each round until you reach 20 repetitions of both the Jump Squat and Superman, or until you can no longer perform the workout.

Notes:

Workout 206:
(Perform 8-10 Rounds)
30 Seconds of Crab Walks
15 Push-ups
30 Seconds of Crab Kicks
15 Tuck Jumps

Notes:

Workout 207:

Starting at minute 0, perform 1 Lunge (each side), followed by rest for the remainder of the minute. At the beginning of the next minute (minute 1), once again perform this process, but add 1 repetition to the exercise. Continue this process, adding 1 repetition to the exercise each round until you reach 20 repetitions of Lunges (each side) or until you can no longer perform the workout.

(2-Minute Rest)

1-Mile Run

Notes:

Workout 208:

(Perform 3-5 Rounds)
5 Chin-ups
30 Seconds of Single-leg Deadlifts
10 Chin-ups
1 Minute of Butt Kicks
15 Chin-ups
2 Minutes of Front Kicks

Notes:

Workout 209:

Starting at minute 0, perform an exercise for 20 seconds, followed by 10 seconds of rest. At the 30-second mark, perform the same exercise another 20 seconds, followed by 10 seconds of rest. Repeat this process a total of 8 times; therefore, you finish at the four-minute mark.

Tabata 1: Plank Reaches
(1-Minute Rest)
Tabata 2: Leg Lifts
(1-Minute Rest)
Tabata 3: Superman Push-ups
(1-Minute Rest)
Tabata 4: Skaters

Notes:

Workout 210:

1-Mile Run

(Then...)
Perform as many Air Squats as you can, followed by Crunches until fatigue. Start again with Air Squats, repeating the process. Continue until you reach 200 Air Squats.

Notes:

Workout 211:
(Perform 5-7 Rounds)
30 Seconds of Bear Crawls
1 Minute of Jump-overs
30 Seconds of Mountain Climbers
1 Minute of Jump-overs

Notes:

Workout 212:
(Perform for 20 Minutes)
30 Leg Lifts
25 Supermans
20 Push-ups
15 Leg Lifts
10 Supermans
5 Push-ups

Notes:

Workout 213:
(Perform for 20 Minutes)
5 Handstand Push-ups
10 Tuck Jumps
30 Seconds of Frozen V Sit

Notes:

Workout 214:
(Perform 8-10 Rounds)
30 Seconds of Inchworms
30 Seconds of Heismans
30 Seconds of Bear Crawls
30 Seconds of Uppercut Punches

Notes:

Workout 215:
(Perform 5-7 Rounds)
2 Minutes of Burpee Push-ups
20 Calf Raises
1 Minute of Punches
20 Dips

Notes:

Workout 216:
(Perform 8-10 Rounds)
15 Pike Push-ups
10 Sit-ups
5 Pull-ups

Notes:

Workout 217:
(Perform for 20 Minutes)
30 Seconds of Butt Kicks
10 Single-leg Deadlifts (each side)
10 Bridges
10 Deadlifts
30 Seconds of Donkey Kicks

Notes:

Workout 218:
(Perform 3-5 Rounds)
4-Minute Run
30 Push-ups
15 Calf Raises

Notes:

Workout 219:
Starting at minute 0, perform 1 Tuck Jump, followed by 1 Chin-up, followed by rest for the remainder of the minute. At the beginning of the next minute (minute 1), once again perform this process, but add 1 repetition to both exercises. Continue this process, adding 1 repetition to both exercises each round until you reach 20 repetitions of both the Tuck Jump and Chin-up, or until you can no longer perform the workout.

Notes:

Workout 220:
(Perform 5-7 Rounds)
1 Minute of Wall Squat
30 Seconds of Plank
1 Minute of Burpees
30 Seconds of Plank

Notes:

Workout 221:
1-Mile Run
2 Minutes of Foot-to-foot Crunches
1-Mile Run
2 Minutes of Bicycles
1-Mile Run

Notes:

Workout 222:
(Perfrom 1-3 Rounds)
1 Minute of Heismans
100 Reverse Flyes
1 Minute of Heismans
75 Calf Raises
1 Minute of Heismans
50 Supermans
1 Minute of Heismans
25 Broad Jumps

Notes:

Workout 223:
(Perform for 20 Minutes)
20 Wipers (side-to-side is 1)
30 Seconds of Crunches
1 Minute of Jumping Jacks

Notes:

Workout 224:
Starting at minute 0, perform an exercise for 20 seconds, followed by 10 seconds of rest. At the 30-second mark, perform the same exercise another 20 seconds, followed by 10 seconds of rest. Repeat this process a total of 8 times; therefore, you finish at the four-minute mark.

Tabata 1: Staggered Push-ups
(1-Minute Rest)
Tabata 2: Skaters
(1-Minute Rest)
Tabata 3: Hindu Push-ups
(1-Minute Rest)
Tabata 4: Climbers

Notes:

Workout 225:
3 Minutes of Sit-ups
15 Pull-ups followed by 1 Lunge (each side)
14 Pull-ups followed by 2 Lunges (each side)
And so on…until you complete 1 Pull-up followed by 15 Lunges (each side)
3 Minutes of Sit-ups

Notes:

Workout 226:
(Perform 3-5 Rounds)
1 Minute of Burpee Broad Jumps
30 Seconds of Dragon Walks
1 Minute of Bicycles
30 Seconds of Dragon Walks
1 Minute of Flutter Kicks
30 Seconds of Dragon Walks

Notes:

Workout 227:
(Perform 5-7 Rounds)
10 Inchworm Push-ups
1 Minute of Kickbacks
5 Burpee Push-ups
1 Minute of Front Kicks

Notes:

Workout 228:
Starting at minute 0, perform 15 Deadlifts, followed by Pike Push-ups for the remainder of the minute. At the beginning of the next minute (minute 1) once again perform 15 Deadlifts, followed by Pike Push-ups for the remainder of the minute. Continue this process until you reach 100 Pike Push-ups.

Notes:

Workout 229:
(Perform for 20 Minutes)
400-Meter Run
20 Wide Push-ups
10 Diamond Push-ups

Notes:

Workout 230:
(Perform for 20 Minutes)
10 Air Squats
8 Supermans
6 Lunges (each side)
4 Inchworms
2 Wall Walks

Notes:

Workout 231:
(Perform 1-3 Rounds)
10 Incline Push-ups followed by 15 Seconds of Frozen V Sit
9 Incline Push-ups followed by 15 Seconds of Frozen V Sit
And so on...until you complete 1 Incline Push-up followed by
15 Seconds of Frozen V Sit
30 Seconds of Right-side Plank Twists
30 Seconds of Left-side Plank Twists

Notes:

Workout 232:
(Perform 8-10 Rounds)
30 Seconds of Bear Crawls
30 Seconds of Broad Jumps
30 Seconds of Dragon Walks
30 Seconds of Tuck Jumps

Notes:

Workout 233:
1 Minute of Plank Jumps
1 Minute of Single-leg Deadlifts
150 Sit-ups
1 Minute of Plank Jumps
1 Minute of Single-leg Deadlifts
1-Mile Run

Notes:

Workout 234:
(Perform for 20 Minutes)
20 Reverse Flyes
20 Plank Reaches (each side)
20 Supermans
20 Leg Lifts
15 Reverse Flyes
15 Plank Reaches (each side)
15 Supermans
15 Leg Lifts
10 Reverse Flyes
10 Plank Reaches (each side)
10 Supermans
10 Leg Lifts
5 Reverse Flyes
5 Plank Reaches (each side)
5 Supermans
5 Leg Lifts

Notes:

Workout 235:
(Perform for 20 Minutes)
10 Push-ups
30 Seconds of Wall Squat

Notes:

Workout 236:
(Perform 8-10 Rounds)
20 Donkey Kicks (each side)
20 Calf Raises
20 Bridges
20 Plank Jumping Jacks

Notes:

Workout 237:
(Perform 8-10 Rounds)
5 Wall Walks
1 Minute of Climbers
5 Handstand Push-ups
1 Minute of Step-ups

Notes:

Workout 238:
(Perform 8-10 Rounds)
30 Seconds of Butt Kicks
30 Seconds of Punches
30 Seconds of Toy Soldiers
30 Seconds of Uppercut Punches

Notes:

Workout 239:
(Perform for 20 Minutes)
10 Chin-ups
20 Air Squats
30 Seconds of Crunches

Notes:

Workout 240:
(Perform 1-3 Rounds)
30 Seconds of Right-side Plank
1 Hindu Push-up followed by 1 Jump Squat
2 Hindu Push-ups followed by 2 Jump Squats
3 Hindu Push-ups followed by 3 Jump Squats
4 Hindu Push-ups followed by 4 Jump Squats
5 Hindu Push-ups followed by 5 Jump Squats
4 Hindu Push-ups followed by 4 Jump Squats
3 Hindu Push-ups followed by 3 Jump Squats
2 Hindu Push-ups followed by 2 Jump Squats
1 Hindu Push-up followed by 1 Jump Squat
30 Seconds of Left-side Plank

Notes

Workout 241:
(Perform 8-10 Rounds)
15 Deadlifts
30 Seconds of Right-side Shuffles
15 Knee Lifts
30 Seconds of Left-side Shuffles

Notes:

Workout 242:
Starting at minute 0, perform the exercise for 20 seconds, followed by 10 seconds of rest. At the 30-second mark, perform the same exercise another 20 seconds, followed by 10 seconds of rest. Repeat this process a total of 8 times; therefore, you finish at the 4-minute mark.

Tabata 1: Plank Jumps
(1-Minute Rest)
Tabata 2: High Knees
(1-Minute Rest)
Tabata 3: Pull-ups
(1-Minute Rest)
Tabata 4: Butt Kicks

Notes:

Workout 243:
(Perform 3-5 Rounds)
1 Minute of Front Kicks
1 Minute of Side-to-side Hops
1 Minute of Kickbacks
1 Minute of Heismans

Notes:

Workout 244:
Starting at minute 0, perform 1 Superman Push-up, followed by 1 Superman, followed by rest for the remainder of the minute. At the beginning of the next minute (minute 1), once again perform this process, but add 1 repetition to both exercises. Continue this process, adding 1 repetition to both exercises each round until you reach 20 repetitions of both the Superman Push-up and Superman, or until you can no longer perform the workout.

Notes:

Workout 245:
(Perform 5-7 Rounds)
30 seconds of Windmills
30 Seconds of Punches
30 Seconds of Right-side Plank
30 Seconds of Deadlifts
30 Seconds of Uppercut Punches
30 Seconds of Left-side Plank

Notes:

Workout 246:
(Perform for 20 Minutes)
30 Seconds of Frozen V Sit
15 Seconds of Tuck Jumps
(15-Second Rest)

Notes:

Workout 247:
(Perform 8-10 Rounds)
20 Push-ups
20 Lunges (each side)
1 Minute of Mountain Climbers

Notes:

Workout 248:
(Perform 3-5 Rounds)
800-Meter Run
50 Jumping Jacks

Notes:

Workout 249:
50 Calf Raises
40 Burpees
30 Wipers (side-to-side is 1)
20 Burpees
10 Push-ups
5 Burpees
10 Push-ups
20 Burpees
30 Wipers (side-to-side is 1)
40 Burpees
50 Calf Raises

Notes:

Workout 250:
(Perform 8-10 Rounds)
15 Pike Push-ups
15 Bridges
1 Minute of Crab Kicks

Notes:

Workout 251:
(Perform 3-5 Rounds)
10 Chin-ups
2 Jump-overs (front-to-back is 1)
8 Chin-ups
4 Jump-overs (front-to-back is 1)
6 Chin-ups
6 Jump-overs (front-to-back is 1)
4 Chin-ups
8 Jump-overs (front-to-back is 1)
2 Chin-ups
10 Jump-overs (front-to-back is 1)

Notes:

Workout 252:
(Perform 8-10 Rounds)
10 Decline Push-ups
1 Minute of Bicycles
10 Incline Push-ups
1 Minute of Crunches

Notes:

Workout 253:
Starting at minute 0, perform 45 Seconds of Butt Kicks, followed by rest for the remainder of the minute. At the beginning of the next minute (minute 1), perform Tuck Jumps for the entire minute. Repeat this process until you reach 100 Tuck Jumps.

Notes:

Workout 254:
(Perform 3-5 Rounds)
30 Seconds of Mountain Climbers
1 Burpee Sit-up followed by 1 Dip
2 Burpee Sit-ups followed by 2 Dips
3 Burpee Sit-ups followed by 3 Dips
4 Burpee Sit-ups followed by 4 Dips
5 Burpee Sit-ups followed by 5 Dips
4 Burpee Sit-ups followed by 4 Dips
3 Burpee Sit-ups followed by 3 Dips
2 Burpee Sit-ups followed by 2 Dips
1 Burpee Sit-up followed by 1 Dip

Notes:

Workout 255:
(Perform for 20 Minutes)
30 Seconds of Donkey Kicks
20 Leg Lifts
30 Deadlifts
20 Leg Lifts
30 Seconds of Crab Kicks

Notes:

Workout 256:
100-Meter Run followed by 40 Air Squats
200-Meter Run followed by 30 Air Squats
300-Meter Run followed by 20 Air Squats
400-Meter Run followed by 10 Air Squats
400-Meter Run followed by 10 Air Squats
300-Meter Run followed by 20 Air Squats
200-Meter Run followed by 30 Air Squats
100-Meter Run followed by 40 Air Squats

Notes:

Workout 257:
(Perform 5-7 Rounds)
30 Seconds of Dragon Walks
30 Seconds of Plank
30 Seconds of Bear Crawls
30 Seconds of Plank
30 Seconds of Crab Walks
30 Seconds of Plank

Notes:

Workout 258:
(Perform for 20 Minutes)
1 Minute of Broad Jumps
30 Seconds of Right-side Plank
1 Minute of Side-to-side Hops
30 Seconds of Left-side Plank
1 Minute of Bicycles

Notes:

Workout 259:
(Perform 3-5 Rounds)
30 Reverse Flyes
30 Seconds of Front Kicks
30 Seconds of Kickbacks
30 Supermans
30 Seconds of Front Kicks
30 Seconds of Kickbacks

Notes:

Workout 260:
(Perform 1-3 Rounds)
2 Handstand Push-ups
4 Superman Push-ups
6 Lunges (each side)
8 Jump Squats
10 Pike Push-ups
8 Jump Squats
6 Lunges (each side)
4 Superman Push-ups
2 Handstand Push-ups
400-Meter Run

Notes:

Workout 261:
3 Minutes of Burpee Sit-ups
(1-Minute Rest)
50 Calf Raises
50 Push-ups
1 Minute of Burpee Sit-ups
50 Push-ups
50 Calf Raises
(1-Minute Rest)
3 Minutes of Burpee Sit-ups

Notes:

Workout 262:
(Perform 8-10 Rounds)
12 Lunges (each side)
9 Chin-ups
6 Donkey Kicks (each side)
3 Handstand Push-ups

Notes:

Workout 263:
(Perform 3-5 Rounds)
1 Minute of Inchworms
5 Diamond Push-ups
1 Minute of Side-to-side Hops
10 Wide Push-ups
1 Minute of Mountain Climbers
5 Diamond Push-ups
1 Minute of Jumping Jacks
10 Wide Push-ups

Notes:

Workout 264:
Starting at minute 0, perform 30 Seconds of Plank, followed by rest for the remainder of the minute. At the beginning of the next minute (minute 1), perform Bridges for the entire minute. Repeat this process until you reach 150 Bridges.

Notes:

Workout 265:
(Perform for 20 Minutes)
5 Pike Push-ups
30 Seconds of Heismans
5 Pike Push-ups
30 Seconds of Climbers

Notes:

Workout 266:
(Perform for 20 Minutes)
1 Minute of Plank Jumping Jacks
1 Minute of Skaters
50 Jumping Jacks

Notes:

Workout 267:
(Perform 1-3 Rounds)
50 Sit-ups
40 Air Squats
30 Plank Jumps
20 Leg Lifts
10 Single-leg Deadlifts (each side)

Notes:

Workout 268:
(Perform 5-7 Rounds)
30 Seconds of Plank Reaches
30 Seconds of Push-ups
30 Seconds of Right-side Plank Twists
30 Seconds of Left-side Plank Twists
30 Seconds of Jumping Jacks
30 Seconds of Reverse Flyes

Notes:

Workout 269:
(Perform 8-10 Rounds)
2-Minute Run
30 Seconds of Crunches

Notes:

Workout 270 :
(Perform 8-10 Rounds)
30 Seconds of Wall Squat
1 Minute of Jump-overs
30 Seconds of Air Squats
1 Minute of Side-to-side Hops

Notes:

Workout 271:
(Perform for 20 Minutes)
20 Supermans
10 Decline Push-ups
40 Reverse Flyes
10 Incline Push-ups

Notes:

Workout 272:
Starting at minute 0, perform 3 Handstand Push-ups, followed by 15 Knee Lifts, followed by rest for the remainder of the minute. At the beginning of the next minute (minute 1), perform 3 Handstand Push-ups, followed by 15 Knee Lifts, followed by rest for the remainder of the minute. Repeat this process until you reach 20 Minutes of working out.

Notes:

Workout 273:
50 Tuck Jumps
15 Pull-ups followed by 1 Tuck Jump
14 Pull-ups followed by 2 Tuck Jumps
And so on...until you complete 1 Pull-up followed by 15 Tuck Jumps
2 Minutes of Pull-ups

Notes:

Workout 274:

Starting at minute 0, perform the exercise for 20 seconds, followed by 10 seconds of rest. At the 30-second mark, perform the same exercise another 20 seconds, followed by 10 seconds of rest. Repeat this process a total of 8 times; therefore, you finish at the 4-minute mark.

Tabata 1: Lunges
(1-Minute Rest)
Tabata 2: Pike Reaches
(1-Minute Rest)
Tabata 3: Plank Jumps
(1-Minute Rest)
Tabata 4: Pike Push-up

Notes:

Workout 275:

(Perform for 20 Minutes)
7 Push-ups followed by 7 Burpee Sit-ups
5 Incline Push-ups followed by 5 Burpee Sit-ups
3 Decline Push-ups followed by 3 Burpee Sit-ups

Notes:

Workout 276:
(Perform 8-10 Rounds)
30 Seconds of Windmills
30 Seconds of Mountain Climbers
30 Seconds of Uppercut Punches
20 Broad Jumps

Notes:

Workout 277:
(Perform 1-3 Rounds)
10 Pike Push-ups followed by 10 Leg Lifts
9 Pike Push-ups followed by 9 Leg Lifts
And so on...until you complete 1 Pike Push-up followed by 1 Leg Lift
30 Seconds of Inchworms
1 Minute of Knee Lifts

Notes:

Workout 278:
(Perform 3-5 Rounds)
15 Burpees
1 Minute of Flutter Kicks
1 Minute of Wall Squat
1 Minute of Bicycles

Notes:

Workout 279:
(Perform for 20 Minutes)
15 Seconds of Right-side Plank Twists
15 Seconds of Left-side Plank Twists
15 Seconds of Plank
(15-Second Rest)

Notes:

Workout 280:
(Perform for 20 Minutes)
5 Superman Push-ups
10 Step-ups
15 Staggered Push-ups
20 Tuck Jumps

Notes:

Workout 281:
(Perform for 20 Minutes)
1 Pull-up
2 Inchworms
3 Air Squats
2 Pull-ups
4 Inchworms
6 Air Squats
3 Pull-ups
6 Inchworms
9 Air Squats

Notes:

Workout 282:
150 Burpee Broad Jumps or Burpee Broad Jumps for 20 Minutes, whichever comes first

Notes:

Workout 283:
(Perform for 20 Minutes)
1 Minute of Leg Lifts
30 Incline Push-ups
30 Crunches
25 Push-ups
25 Sit-ups
20 Decline Push-ups
20 Knee Lifts
15 Incline Push-ups
15 Crunches
10 Push-ups
10 Sit-ups
5 Decline Push-ups
5 Knee Lifts
1 Minute of Hindu Push-ups

Notes:

Workout 284:
5-Minute Run
30 Seconds of Air Squats
4-Minute Run
30 Seconds of Air Squats
3-Minute Run
30 Seconds of Air Squats
2-Minute Run
30 Seconds of Air Squats
1-Minute Run
30 Seconds of Air Squats

Notes:

Workout 285:
(Perform for 20 Minutes)
15 Jump-overs (front-to-back is 1) followed by 15 Deadlifts
14 Jump-overs (front-to-back is 1) followed by 14 Deadlifts
And so on...until you complete 1 Jump-over followed by 1 Deadlift

Notes:

Workout 286:
1 Minute of Push-ups
10 Supermans followed by 1 Hindu Push-up
9 Supermans followed by 2 Hindu Push-ups
And so on...until you complete 1 Superman followed by 10 Hindu Push-ups
50 Reverse Flyes
40 Push-ups
30 Reverse Flyes
20 Push-ups
10 Reverse Flyes

Notes:

Workout 287:

Starting at minute 0, perform an exercise for 20 seconds, followed by 10 seconds of rest. At the 30-second mark, perform the same exercise another 20 seconds, followed by 10 seconds of rest. Repeat this process a total of 8 times; therefore, you finish at the 4-minute mark.

Tabata 1: Shuffles (switch side every 20 seconds)
(1-Minute Rest)
Tabata 2: Jump Squats
(1-Minute Rest)
Tabata 3: Side-to-side Hops
(1-Minute Rest)
Tabata 4: Toe Touches

Notes:

Workout 288:

(Perform 8-10 Rounds)
30 Seconds of Burpees
30 Seconds of Flutter Kicks
30 Seconds of Wide Push-ups
30 Seconds of Bicycles

Notes:

Workout 289:
(Perform for 20 Minutes)
15 Seconds of Right-side Plank
15 Seconds of Left-side Plank
15 Seconds of Jump Squats
(15-Second Rest)

Notes:

Workout 290:
(Perform for 20 Minutes)
5 Handstand Push-ups
10 Pull-ups
15 Single-leg Deadlifts (each side)

Notes:

Workout 291:
(Perform for 20 Minutes)
20 Broad Jumps
15 Push-ups
5 Burpees

Notes:

The Workouts

Workout 292:
(Perform 5-7 Rounds)
30 Seconds of Right-side Shuffles
30 Seconds of Plank
30 Seconds of Bridges
30 Seconds of High Knees
30 Seconds of Bridges
30 Seconds of Plank
30 Seconds of Left-side Shuffles

Notes:

Workout 293:
(Perform for 20 Minutes)
10 Deadlifts
10 Inchworms
10 Air Squats
10 Pike Push-ups

Notes:

Workout 294:
(Perform 1-3 Rounds)
12 Push-ups followed by 30 Seconds of Right-side Shuffles
11 Push-ups followed by 30 Seconds of Left-side Shuffles
And so on...until you complete 1 Push-up followed by 30 Seconds of Left-side Shuffles

Notes:

Workout 295:
(Perform 5-7 Rounds)
1 Minute of Front Kicks
30 Plank Jumps
30 Calf Raises
30 Plank Jumping Jacks
1 Minute of Kickbacks

Notes:

Workout 296:
(Perform 3-5 Rounds)
1 Minute of Crunches
20 Lunges (each side)
1 Minute of Toe Touches
20 Single-leg Deadlifts (each side)
1 Minute of Jumping Jacks

Notes:

Workout 297:
50 Burpee Push-ups
(2-Minute Rest)
15-Minute Run

Notes:

Workout 298:
50 Pull-ups
1-Mile Run
50 Supermans
1-Mile run
50 Reverse Flyes

Notes:

Workout 299:
(Perform 8-10 Rounds)
30 Seconds of Crab Walks
30 Seconds of Bear Crawls

(1-Minute Rest, then...)
3 Minutes of Side-to-side Hops
2 Minutes of Wall Squat
1 Minute of Skaters
30 Seconds of Plank

Notes:

Workout 300:
Starting at minute 0, perform 1 minute of Heismans for the entire minute. At the beginning of the next minute (minute 1), perform Sit-ups for the entire minute. Repeat this process until you reach 150 Sit-ups.

Notes:

Workout 301:
(Perform 3-5 Rounds)
2 Minutes of Punches
15 Calf Raises
1 Minute of Mountain Climbers
15 Calf Raises
30 Seconds of Climbers
15 Calf Raises

Notes:

Workout 302:
(Perform for 20 Minutes)
1 Minute of Crab Kicks
10 Air Squats followed by 10 Pull-ups
9 Air Squats followed by 9 Pull-ups
And so on...until you complete 1 Air Squat followed by 1 Pull-up

Notes:

Workout 303:

Starting at minute 0, perform an exercise for 20 seconds, followed by 10 seconds of rest. At the 30-second mark, perform the same exercise another 20 seconds, followed by 10 seconds of rest. Repeat this process a total of 8 times; therefore, you finish at the four-minute mark.

Tabata 1: Wipers
(1-Minute Rest)
Tabata 2: Staggered Push-ups
(1-Minute Rest)
Tabata 3: Foot-to-foot Crunches
(1-Minute Rest)
Tabata 4: Toy Soldiers

Notes:

Workout 304:

(Perform 1-3 Rounds)
10 Inchworm Push-ups
20 Deadlifts
30 Jump Squats
40 Step-ups
50 Air Squats

Notes:

THE WORKOUTS

Workout 305:
(Perform for 20 Minutes)
30 Burpees
1 Minute of Plank Reaches
30 Supermans

Notes:

Workout 306:
(Perform for 20 Minutes)
30 Seconds of Butt Kicks
30 Seconds of High Knees
30 Seconds of Uppercut Punches
15 Plank Jumping Jacks
10 Tuck Jumps
5 Plank Jumps

Notes:

Workout 307:
(Perform 3-5 Rounds)
1 Minute of Crunches
10 Pull-ups
1 Minute of Leg Lifts
10 Chin-ups
1 Minute of Knee Lifts
10 Pull-ups

Notes:

Workout 308:
(Perform for 20 Minutes)
50 Air Squats
1 Minute of Pike Push-ups
1 Minute of Mountain Climbers

Notes:

Workout 309:
(Perform 8-10 Rounds)
30 Seconds of Tuck Jumps
30 Seconds of Plank Jumping Jacks
30 Seconds of Jumping Jacks
30 Seconds of Crab Kicks

Notes:

Workout 310:
(Perform 5-7 Rounds)
1 Minute of Skaters
5 Inchworms
1 Minute of Foot-to-foot Crunches
5 Inchworms
1 Minute of Heismans
5 Inchworms

Notes:

Workout 311:
(Perform 8-10 Rounds)
30 Seconds of Right-side Shuffles
10 Burpee Push-ups
30 Seconds of Left-side Shuffles

Notes:

Workout 312:
(Perform 3-5 Rounds)
1 Minute of Toy Soldiers
30 Seconds of Frozen V Sit
1 Minute of Donkey Kicks
30 Seconds of Frozen V Sit
1 Minute of Climbers
30 Seconds of Frozen V Sit

Notes:

Workout 313:
(Perform 5-7 Rounds)
15 Single-leg Deadlifts (each leg)
15 Sit-ups
15 Windmills (side-to-side is 1)
15 Leg Lifts

Notes:

Workout 314:
100-Meter Run followed by 40 Push-ups
200-Meter Run followed by 30 Push-ups
300-Meter Run followed by 20 Push-ups
400-Meter Run followed by 10 Push-ups
300-Meter Run followed by 20 Push-ups
200-Meter Run followed by 30 Push-ups
100-Meter Run followed by 40 Push-ups

Notes:

Workout 315:
Starting at minute 0, perform an exercise for 20 seconds, followed by 10 seconds of rest. At the 30-second mark, perform the same exercise another 20 seconds, followed by 10 seconds of rest. Repeat this process a total of 8 times; therefore, you finish at the 4-minute mark.

Tabata 1: Reverse Flyes
(1-Minute Rest)
Tabata 2: Right-side Plank Twists
(1-Minute Rest)
Tabata 3: Left-side Plankt Twists
(1-Minute Rest)
Tabata 4: Plank

Notes:

Workout 316:
(Perform for 20 Minutes)
1 Minute of Bicycles
30 Seconds of Crab Walks
50 Sit-ups
30 Seconds of Bear Crawls
1 Minute of Crunches

Notes:

Workout 317:
(Perform 5-7 Rounds)
1 Minute of Mountain Climbers
30 Plank Jumping Jacks
1 Minute of Heismans
30 Plank Jumping Jacks

Notes:

Workout 318:
10 Wide Push-ups followed by 1 Tuck Jump
9 Wide Push-ups followed by 2 Tuck Jumps
And so on...until you complete 1 Wide Push-up followed by
10 Tuck Jumps
15-Minute Run

Notes:

Workout 319:
(Perform for 20 Minutes)
30 Seconds of Dragon Walks
30 Seconds of Sit-ups
30 Broad Jumps
30 Seconds of Bear Crawls
30 Seconds of Crunches
30 Broad Jumps

Notes:

Workout 320:
Starting at minute 0, perform 1 Burpee, followed by 1 Chin-up, followed by rest for the remainder of the minute. At the beginning of the next minute (minute 1), once again perform this process, but add 1 repetition to both exercises.
Continue this process, adding 1 repetition to both exercises each round until you reach 20 repetitions of both the Burpee and Chin-up, or until you can no longer perform the workout.

Notes:

Workout 321:
(Perform 3-5 Rounds)
30 Seconds of Wall Squat
1 Minute of Jump-overs

(1-Minute of Rest, then...)
(Perform 3-5 Rounds)
20 Lunges (each side)
30 Seconds of Inchworms

Notes:

Workout 322:
(Perform 3-5 Rounds)
30 Seconds of Crab Walks
10 Decline Push-ups
30 Seconds of Climbers
10 Dips
30 Seconds of Heismans
10 Incline Push-ups

Notes:

Workout 323:
2 Minutes of Burpees
50 Windmills (side-to-side is 1)
50 Kickbacks (each side)
40 Windmills (side-to-side is 1)
40 Kickbacks (each side)
30 Windmills (side-to-side is 1)
30 Kickbacks (each side)
20 Windmills (side-to-side is 1)
20 Kickbacks (each side)
10 Windmills (side-to-side is 1)
10 Kickbacks (each side)
2 Minutes of Burpees

Notes:

Workout 324:
1-Mile Run
50 Jumping Jacks
40 Plank Jumping Jacks
30 Side-to-side Hops
20 Jump Squats
10 Tuck Jumps
1-Mile Run

Notes:

Workout 325:
(Perform 1-3 Rounds)
50 Air Squats
40 Wide Push-ups
30 Seconds Frozen V Sit
20 Lunges (each leg)
10 Diamond Push-ups

Notes:

Workout 326:
(Perform 5-7 Rounds)
30 Seconds of Plank
10 Sit-ups
30 Seconds of Front Kicks
10 Sit-ups
30 Seconds of Toy Soldiers
10 Sit-ups
30 Seconds of Punches
10 Sit-ups

Notes:

Workout 327:
Starting at minute 0, perform 1 Pike Push-up, followed by 1 Air Squat, followed by rest for the remainder of the minute. At the beginning of the next minute (minute 1), once again perform this process, but add 1 repetition to both exercises. Continue this process, adding 1 repetition to both exercises each round until you reach 20 repetitions of both the Pike Push-up and Air Squat, or until you can no longer perform the workout.

Notes:

Workout 328:
(Perform for 20 Minutes)
400-Meter Run
10 Supermans
20 Leg Lifts
30 Reverse Flyes

Notes:

Workout 329:
(Perform 1-3 Rounds)
3 Minutes of Side-to-side Hops
2 Minutes of Burpee Broad Jumps
1 Minute of Dragon Walk
30 Seconds of Frozen V Sit

Notes:

Workout 330:
Starting at minute 0, perform an exercise for 20 seconds, followed by 10 seconds of rest. At the 30-second mark, perform the same exercise another 20 seconds, followed by 10 seconds of rest. Repeat this process a total of 8 times; therefore, you finish at the 4-minute mark.

Tabata 1: Inchworm Push-ups
(1-Minute Rest)
Tabata 2: Chin-ups
(1-Minute of Rest)
Tabata 3: Plank Reaches
(1-Minute Rest)
Tabata 4: Hindu Push-ups

Notes:

Workout 331:
(Perform 1-3 Rounds)
30 Seconds of Right-side Plank Twists
30 Seconds of Left-side Plank Twists
3 Minutes of Jumping Jacks
2 Minutes of Toy Soldiers
1 Minute of Plank

Notes:

Workout 332:
3 Minutes of Crunches
2-Mile Run
3 Minutes of Knee Lifts

Notes

Workout 333:
(Perform for 20 Minutes)
15 Seconds of Air Squats
15 Seconds of Push-ups
15 Seconds of Pull-ups
(15-Second Rest)

Notes:

Workout 334:
(Perform 8-10 Rounds)
30 Seconds of Deadlifts
30 Seconds of Crab Walks
30 Seconds of Toy Soldiers
30 Seconds of Crab Kicks

Notes:

THE WORKOUTS

Workout 335:
(Perform 8-10 Rounds)
30 Seconds of Crunches
10 Pull-ups
10 Supermans
30 Seconds of Bicycles

Notes:

Workout 336:
(Perform for 20 Minutes)
5 Incline Push-ups
5 Air Squats
10 Decline Push-ups
10 Lunges (each side)

Notes:

Workout 337:
(Perform 3-5 Rounds)
1 Minute of Mountain Climbers
30 Seconds of Plank
1 Minute of Kickbacks
30 Seconds of Right-side Plank
1 Minute of Front Kicks
30 Seconds of Left-side Plank

Notes:

Workout 338:
(Perform 1-3 Rounds)
1 Minute of Punches
800-Meter Run
1 Minute of Uppercut Punches
800-Meter Run

Notes:

Workout 339:
(Perform 8-10 Rounds)
5 Handstand Push-ups
20 Jump Squats
30 Seconds of Crab Walks

Notes:

Workout 340:
10 Burpees followed by 1 Inchworm
9 Burpees followed by 2 Inchworms
And so on...until you complete 1 Burpee followed by 10 Inchworms
2 Minutes of Burpees
1 Minute of Inchworms
30 Seconds of Burpees

Notes:

Workout 341:

Starting at minute 0, perform 10 Chin-ups, followed by rest the remainder of the minute. At the beginning of the next minute (minute 1), perform as many Windmills (side-to-side is 1) as you can. Continue this process until you reach 150 Windmills (side-to-side is 1).

Notes:

Workout 342:

(Perform for 20 Minutes)
15 Decline Push-ups followed by 15 Wipers (side-to-side is 1)
14 Decline Push-ups followed by 14 Wipers (side-to-side is 1)
And so on...until you complete 1 Decline Push-up followed by 1 Wiper (side-to-side is 1)

Notes:

Workout 343:

(Perform 5-7 Rounds)
10 Broad Jumps
30 Seconds of Right-side Plank Twists
10 Plank Jumps
30 Seconds of Left-side Plank Twists
10 Tuck Jumps

Notes:

Workout 344:
(Perform for 20 Minutes)
20 Reverse Flyes
15 Toe Touches
10 Supermans
5 Sit-ups

Notes:

Workout 345
Starting at minute 0, perform 15 Hindu Push-ups, followed by rest the remainder of the minute. At the beginning of the next minute (minute 1), perform as many Wipers as you can. Repeat this process until you reach 100 Wipers (side-to-side is 1).

Notes:

Workout 346:
(Perform for 20 Minutes)
30 Step-ups (Even Minutes – 0, 2, and so on...)
30 Side-to-side Hops (Odd Minutes – 1, 3, and so on...)

Notes:

Workout 347:
(Perform 1-3 Rounds)
50 Deadlifts
40 Jumping Jacks
30 Windmills (side-to-side is 1)
20 Plank Jumping Jacks
10 Single-leg Dedlifts (each side)
1 Minute of Punches

Notes:

Workout 348:
(Perform for 20 Minutes)
10 Pike Push-ups followed by 1 Calf Raise
9 Pike Push-ups followed by 2 Calf Raises
And so on...until you complete 1 Pike Push-up followed by 10 Calf Raises
Notes:

Workout 349:
(Perform 8-10 Rounds)
1 Minute of Plank Jumps
1 Minute of Burpee Sit-ups

Notes:

Workout 350:
3 Minutes of Foot-to-foot Crunches
3 Minutes of Leg Lifts
3 Minute of Sit-ups
(2-Minute Rest)
3 Minute of Sit-ups
3 Minutes of Leg Lifts
3 Minutes of Foot-to-foot Crunches

Notes:

Workout 351:
(Perform for 20 Minutes)
15 Seconds of Pull-ups
15 seconds of Toy Soldiers
15 Seconds of Dips
(15-Second Rest)

Notes:

Workout 352:
Starting at minute 0, perform 30 Seconds of Frozen V Sit, followed by rest for the remainder of the minute. At the beginning of the next minute (minute 1), perform Inchworms for the entire minute. Continue this process until you reach 100 Inchworms.

Notes:

Workout 353:
(Perform for 20 Minutes)
30 Seconds of Wall Squat
30 Seconds of Skaters
30 Seconds of Donkey Kicks
30 Seconds of Bear Crawls

Notes:

Workout 354:
(Perform for 20 Minutes)
5 Air Squats
5 Push-ups
10 Air Squats
10 Push-ups
20 Air Squats
20 Push-ups
30 Air Squats
30 Push-ups
100 Reverse Flyes
30 Air Squats
30 Push-ups
20 Air Squats
20 Push-ups
10 Air Squats
10 Push-ups
5 Air Squats
5 Push-ups

Notes:

Workout 355:
(Perform 3-5 Rounds)
800-Meter Run
30 Seconds of Wipers
30 Seconds of Toy Soldiers

Notes:

Workout 356:
(Perform 8-10 Rounds)
3 Pike Push-ups
6 Jump Squats
9 Dips
12 Bridges

Notes:

Workout 357:

Starting at minute 0, perform the exercise for 20 seconds, followed by 10 seconds of rest. At the 30-second mark, perform the same exercise another 20 seconds, followed by 10 seconds of rest. Repeat this process a total of 8 times; therefore, you finish at the 4-minute mark.

Tabata 1: Lunges
(1-Minute of Rest)
Tabata 2: Push-ups
(1-Minute of Rest)
Tabata 3: Tuck Jumps
(1-Minute of Rest)
Tabata 4: Staggered Push-ups

Notes:

Workout 358:

Starting at minute 0, perform the exercise for 20 seconds, followed by 10 seconds of rest. At the 30-second mark, perform the same exercise another 20 seconds, followed by 10 seconds of rest. Repeat this process a total of 8 times; therefore, you finish at the 4-minute mark.

Tabata 1: Right-side Plank Twists
(1-Minute of Rest)
Tabata 2: Left-side Plank Twists
(1-Minute of Rest)
Tabata 3: Leg Lifts
(1-Minute of Rest)
Tabata 4: Shuffles (switch sides every 20 seconds)

Notes:

Workout 359:
(Perform 8-10 Rounds)
30 Seconds of Push-ups
30 Seconds of Air Squats
30 Seconds of Pull-ups
30 Seconds of Sit-ups

Notes:

Workout 360:
(Perform 8-10 Rounds)
30 Seconds of Crab Walks
10 Single-leg Deadlifts (each side)
30 Seconds of Crab Kicks
20 Windmills (Side-to-side is 1)

Notes:

Workout 361:
(Perform 8-10 Rounds)
5 Jump Squats
10 Jump-overs (front-to-back is 1)
15 Plank Jumping Jacks

Notes:

Workout 362:

50 Burpee Push-ups
1 Minute of Punches
1 Minute of Plank Reaches
150 Jumping Jacks
1 Minute of Plank Reaches
1 Minute of Uppercut Punches
50 Burpee Sit-ups

Notes:

Workout 363:

(Perform 3-5 Rounds)
2 Superman Push-ups
4 Lunges (each leg)
6 Pike Push-ups
8 Air Squats
10 Push-ups
8 Air Squats
6 Pike Push-ups
4 Lunges (each leg)
2 Superman Push-ups

Notes:

Workout 364:

(Perform 8-10 Rounds)
30 Seconds of High Knees
30 Seconds of Dragon Walk
1 Minute of Burpees

Notes:

Workout 365:
1 Minute of Leg Lifts
50 Push-ups
1 Minute of Flutter Kicks
40 Dips
1 Minute of Bicycles
30 Pike Push-ups
1 Minute of Leg Lifts
20 Burpee Push-ups
1 Minute of Flutter Kicks
10 Inchworms
1 Minute of Bicycles

Notes:

AND MORE...
KETTLEBELL
WORKOUTS

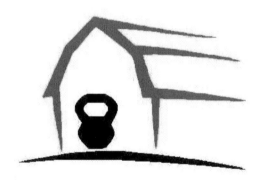

"YOU ARE NEVER TOO OLD TO SET
ANOTHER GOAL OR TO DREAM A NEW
DREAM."

- C. S. LEWIS

THE WORKOUTS

Workout 1:
(Perform 1-3 Rounds)
20 Kettlebell Swings
20 Push-ups
20 Sit-ups
15 Kettlebell Swings
15 Push-ups
15 Sit-ups
10 Kettlebell Swings
10 Push-ups
10 Sit-ups
5 Kettlebell Swings
5 Push-ups
5 Sit-ups

Notes:

Workout 2:
(Perform for 20 Minutes)
10 Kettlebell Front Squats
10 Pull-ups
20 Air Squats
20 Reverse Flyes

Notes:

Workout 3:

Starting at minute 0, perform the exercise for 20 seconds, followed by 10 seconds of rest. At the 30-second mark, perform the same exercise another 20 seconds, followed by 10 seconds of rest. Repeat this process a total of 8 times; therefore, you finish at the 4-minute mark.

Tabata 1: Kettlebell Squat-presses
(1-Minute Rest)
Tabata 2: Crunches
(1-Minute Rest)
Tabata 3: Kettlebell High-pulls
(1-Minute Rest)
Tabata 4: Leg Lifts

Notes:

Workout 4:

(Perform for 20 Minutes)
10 Kettlebell Rows (each side)
1 Minute of Jumping Jacks
10 Supermans
1 Minute of Heismans

Notes:

Workout 5:

Starting at minute 0, perform 10 Kettlebell Deadlifts, followed by Wide Push-ups for the remainder of the minute. At the beginning of the next minute (minute 1), once again perform 10 Kettlebell Deadlifts followed by Wide Push-ups for the remainder of the minute. Continue this process until you reach 100 Wide Push-ups.

Notes:

Workout 6:

(Perform 8-10 Rounds)
15 Broad Jumps
30 Seconds of Bear Crawls
15 Kettlebell Rows (each side)
30 Seconds of Dragon Walks

Notes:

Workout 7:

(Perform 8-10 Rounds)
15 Incline Push-ups
15 Kettlebell Figure-8s
15 Decline Push-ups
15 Wipers (side-to-side is 1)

Notes:

Workout 8:
(Perform for 20 Minutes)
30 Seconds of High Knees
10 Kettlebell High Pulls
30 Seconds of Butt Kicks
10 Kettlebell Swings

Notes:

Workout 9:
Starting at minute 0, perform the exercise for 20 seconds, followed by 10 seconds of rest. At the 30-second mark, perform the same exercise another 20 seconds, followed by 10 seconds of rest. Repeat this process a total of 8 times; therefore, you finish at the 4-minute mark.

Tabata 1: Kettlebell Rows (switch sides every 20 seconds)
(1-Minute Rest)
Tabata 2: Plank Jumps
(1-Minute Rest)
Tabata 3: Pull-ups
(1-Minute Rest)
Tabata 4: Plank Jumping Jacks

Notes:

Workout 10:
(Perform 8-10 Rounds)
10 Kettlebell Push-ups
1 Minute of Uppercut Punches
10 Kettlebell Push-ups
1 Minute of Skaters

Notes:

Workout 11:
(Perform 8-10 Rounds)
10 Kettlebell Around the Worlds
10 Toe Touches
10 Tuck Jumps
10 Calf Raises

Notes:

Workout 12:
Starting at minute 0, perform 30 Seconds of Side-to-side Hops, followed by Kettlebell Deadlifts for the remainder of the minute. At the beginning of the next minute (minute 1), once again perform 30 Seconds of Side-to-side Hops followed by Kettlebell Deadlifts for the remainder of the minute. Continue this process until you reach 100 Kettlebell Deadlifts.

Notes:

Workout 13:
(Perform 1-3 Rounds)
50 Jumping Jacks
40 Leg Lifts
30 Kettlebell Military Presses
20 Burpees
10 Pike Push-ups

Notes:

Workout 14:
(Perform 5-7 Rounds)
20 Lunges (each side)
10 Right-arm Rows
20 Air Squats
10 Left-arm Rows
1 Minute of Jump-overs

Notes:

Workout 15:
(Perform 8-10 Rounds)
30 Seconds of Kettlebell Figure-8s
30 Seconds of Burpee Broad Jumps
30 Seconds of Bicycles
30 Seconds of Climbers

Notes:

Workout 16:
(Perform for 20 Minutes)
15 Kettlebell Front Squats
15 Hindu Push-ups
15 Leg Lifts

Notes:

Workout 17:
(Perform for 20 Minutes)
800-Meter Run
10 Burpees
10 Kettlebell Deadlifts

Notes:

THE WORKOUTS

Workout 18:
Starting at minute 0, perform the exercise for 20 seconds, followed by 10 seconds of rest. At the 30-second mark, perform the same exercise another 20 seconds, followed by 10 seconds of rest. Repeat this process a total of 8 times; therefore, you finish at the 4-minute mark.

Tabata 1: Kettlebell Figure-8s
(1-Minute Rest)
Tabata 2: Toy Soldiers
(1-Minute of Rest)
Tabata 3: Kettlebell Around the Worlds
(1-Minute Rest)
Tabata 4: Step-ups

Notes:

Workout 19:
(Perform 5-7 Rounds)
15 Kettlebell Swings
30 Seconds of Mountain Climbers
30 Seconds of Punches
30 Seconds of Dragon Walks
30 Seconds of Uppercut Punches

Notes:

Workout 20:
(Perform for 20 Minutes)
50 Push-ups
40 Knee Lifts
30 Kettlebell Push-ups
20 Sit-ups
10 Dips

Notes:

Workout 21:
(Perform for 20 Minutes)
10 Kettlebell Front Squats
20 Plank Jumps
30 Leg Lifts

Notes:

Workout 22:
(Perform 5-7 Rounds)
30 Seconds of High Knees
10 Right-arm Rows
30 Seconds of Butt Kicks
10 Left-arm Rows
30 Seconds of Plank
10 Pull-ups

Notes:

Workout 23:
(Perform 5-7 Rounds)
10 Kettlebell High Pulls
30 Seconds of Crab Kicks
30 Seconds of Crunches
10 Kettlebell Military Presses
30 Seconds of Donkey kicks
30 Seconds of Crunches

Notes:

Workout 24:
(Perform for 20 Minutes)
10 Single-leg Deadlifts (each side)
10 Staggered Push-ups
10 Kettlebell Deadlifts
10 Staggered Push-ups
10 Inchworms

Notes:

Workout 25:
(Perform 5-7 Rounds)
20 Supermans
15 Calf Raises
10 Kettlebell Around the Worlds
5 Plank Jumping Jacks
1 Minute of Punches

Notes:

Workout 26:
(Perform 8-10 Rounds)
10 Kettlebell Squat-presses
1 Minute of Climbers
30 Seconds of Crab Walk

Notes:

Workout 27:
Starting at minute 0, perform 30 Seconds of Side-to-side Hops followed by Alternating-arm Kettlebell Rows for the remainder of the minute. At the beginning of the next minute (minute 1), once again perform 30 Seconds of Side-to-side Hops followed by Alternating-arm Kettlebell Rows for the remainder of the minute. Continue this process until you reach 100 Kettlebell Rows (each side).

Notes:

Workout 28:
(Perform for 20 Minutes)
5 Chin-ups
10 Kettlebell Figure-8s
15 Air Squats

Notes:

Workout 29:
(Perform for 20 Minutes)
400-Meter Run
15 Kettlebell Swings

Notes:

Workout 30:
(Perform 8-10 Rounds)
10 Kettlebell Front Squats
30 Seconds of Plank Jumping Jacks
30 Seconds of Windmills
30 Seconds of Punches

Notes:

Workout 31:
(Perform for 20 Minutes)
50 Knee Lifts
40 Burpee Push-ups
30 Sit-ups
20 Kettlebell Push-ups
10 Jump Squats

Notes:

Workout 32:
(Perform 8-10 Rounds)
15 Seconds of Kettlebell Figure-8s
15 Seconds of Toy Soldiers
15 Seconds of Plank
(15-Second Rest)

Notes:

Workout 33:
(Perform for 20 Minutes)
10 Kettlebell High-pulls (Even Minutes – 0, 2, and so on...)
5 Pike Push-ups (Odd Minutes – 1, 3, and so on...)

Notes:

Workout 34:
(Perform for 20 Minutes)
12 Kettlebell Front Squats followed by 30 Seconds of Flutter Kicks
11 Kettlebell Front Squats followed by 30 Seconds of Flutter Kicks
And so on... until you complete 1 Kettlebell Front Squat followed by 30 Seconds of Flutter Kicks

Notes:

Workout 35:
(Perform 3-5 Rounds)
30 Seconds of Left-side Shuffles
10 Kettlebell Rows (each side)
20 Kettlebell Deadlifts
30 Jump-overs
30 Seconds of Right-side Shuffles

Notes:

Workout 36:
(Perform 5-7 Rounds)
7 Kettlebell Around the Worlds followed by 7 Inchworms
followed by 7 Sit-ups
5 Kettlebell Around the Worlds followed by 5 Inchworms
followed by 5 Sit-ups
3 Kettlebell Around the Worlds followed by 3 Inchworms
followed by 3 Sit-ups

Notes:

Workout 37:
(Perform 1-3 Rounds)
20 Kettlebell Deadlifts
20 Incline Push-ups
15 Kettlebell Front Squats
15 Decline Push-ups
10 Kettlebell Deadlifts
10 Incline Push-ups
5 Kettlebell Front Squats
5 Decline Push-ups
30 Seconds of Heismans

Notes:

Workout 38:
(Perform 3-5 Rounds)
30 Seconds of Kettlebell Figure-8s
2 Minutes of Bicycles
1 Minute of Burpees
(30-Second Rest)

Notes:

Workout 39:
(Perform for 20 Minutes)
15 Kettlebell Swings
20 Tuck Jumps
30 Seconds of Side-to-side Hopes

Notes:

Workout 40:

Starting at minute 0, perform the exercise for 20 seconds, followed by 10 seconds of rest. At the 30-second mark, perform the same exercise another 20 seconds, followed by 10 seconds of rest. Repeat this process a total of 8 times; therefore, you finish at the 4-minute mark.

Tabata 1: Kettlebell Push-ups
(1-Minute Rest)
Tabata 2: Toy Soldiers
(1-Minute Rest)
Tabata 3: Staggered Push-ups
(1-Minute Rest)
Tabata 4: Plank Reach

Notes:

Workout 41:

(Perform 5-7 Rounds)
10 Kettlebell Rows (each side)
30 Seconds of Left-side Plank
30 Seconds of Right-side Plank
30 Seconds of Wall Squat
30 Calf Raises

Notes:

Workout 42:
50 Kettlebell Front Squats
40 Supermans
30 Air Squats
20 Chin-ups
10 Lunges (each side)
10-Minute Run

Notes:

Workout 43:
(Perform 3-5 Rounds)
20 Kettlebell Around the Worlds
10 Dips
20 Leg Lifts
10 Dips
20 Crunches
10 Dips
1 Minute of Side-to-side Hops

Notes:

Workout 44:
Starting at minute 0, perform 10 Kettlebell Deadlifts followed by Plank Jumps for the remainder of the minute. At the beginning of the next minute (minute 1), once again perform 10 Kettlebell Deadlifts followed by Plank Jumps for the remainder of the minute. Continue this process until you reach 125 Plank Jumps.

Notes:

Workout 45:
Starting at minute 0, perform 5 Kettlebell Squat-presses, followed by 10 Air Squats, followed by rest for the remainder of the minute. At the beginning of the next minute (minute 1), once again perform 5 Kettlebell Squat-presses, followed by 10 Air Squats, followed by rest for the remainder of the minute. Repeat this process until you have worked out for 20 Minutes.

Notes:

Workout 46:
(Perform 3-5 Rounds)
10 Kettlebell High Pulls
30 Seconds of Front Kicks
10 Kettlebell Military Presses
30 Seconds of Kickbacks
10 Kettlebell Swings
30 Seconds of Uppercut Punches

Notes:

Workout 47:
(Perform for 20 Minutes)
30 Seconds of Kettlebell Figure-8s
1 Minute of Dragon Walks
2 Minutes of Foot-to-foot Crunches

Notes:

Workout 48:
(Perform 3-5 Rounds)
20 Wide Push-ups
20 Kettlebell Squat Presses
10 Diamond Push-ups
10 Kettlebell Squat Presses
(30-Second Rest)

Notes:

Workout 49:
(Perform for 20 Minutes)
10 Kettlebell Push-ups
10 Pull-ups
10 Tuck Jumps

Notes:

Workout 50:
(Perform 1-3 Rounds)
50 Kettlebell Deadlifts
40 Plank Jumping Jacks
30 Kettlebell Swings
20 Burpees
10 Kettlebell Squat Presses

Notes:

INDEX

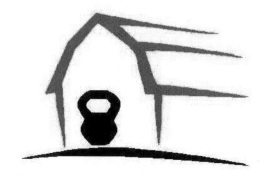

INDEX

INDEX

Run

Shoulders

See Bear Crawl, Burpee, Burpee Broad Jump, Burpee Push-up, Crab Kick, Crab Walk, Decline Push-up, Diamond Push-up, Dip, Dragon Walk, Handstand Push-up, Hindu Push-up, Inchworm, Inchworm Push-up, Incline Push-up, Jumping Jack, Kettlebell Around the World, Kettlebell Deadlift, Kettlebell Figure-8, Kettlebell Front Squat, Kettlebell High Pull, Kettlebell Military Press, Kettlebell Push-up, Kettlebell Row, Kettlebell Swing, Kettlebell Squat Press, Pike Push-up, Plank, Plank Jump, Plank Jumping Jack, Plank Reach, Punch, Push-up, Side Plank, Side Plank Twist, Staggered Push-up, Superman, Superman Push-up, Uppercut Punch, Wall Walk, Wide Push-up

Shuffle

Side Plank

Side Plank Twist

Side-to-side Hop

INDEX

ABOUT THE AUTHOR

Farmer Gym founder Jason Harle is certified through the American Council on Exercise. He is an ACE-Certified Personal Trainer and an ACE-Certified Health Coach; he is also a CrossFit Level-1 Trainer. Coach Harle has worked as a collegiate strength and conditioning coach, has developed and managed a track and cross country academic research journal, and has taught as a collegiate sports and fitness professor. In developing Farmer Gym, Coach Harle has drawn on the ideas of various exercise regimens and theories, and united them with the type of work found in a farmer's way of life.

Coach Harle resides in Pacific Palisades, California, with his wife, Denise Mayo Harle. He trains clients online, providing personalized fitness programs designed to advance the particular health and wellness goals of each of Farmer Gym's clients. Coach Harle's mission for Farmer Gym is to educate, motivate, and empower others to live lives of improved, sustainable health.